Fitness Journal

Fitness Journal

Patrick P. Stack

iUniverse, Inc.
New York Lincoln Shanghai

Fitness Journal

iUniverse, Inc.

For information address:
iUniverse, Inc.
2021 Pine Lake Road, Suite 100
Lincoln, NE 68512
www.iuniverse.com

ISBN: 0-595-30567-9

Printed in the United States of America

Contents

INTRODUCTION

Why is it so important to keep a Fitness Journal?

- A fitness journal will help you analyze all facets of the three most vital ingredients in fitness.

  These important principals to follow in order to attain your peak physical fitness are:

  - ➢ NUTRITION/DIET
  - ➢ REGULAR EXERCISE
  - ➢ SLEEP (muscle recovery is 48 hours)

- A fitness journal helps you track your workouts and eating habits more efficiently.

- A fitness journal offers you insight into your own strengths and weaknesses in regards to your fitness and nutrition regime. You can then use this new insight to modify your training/diet in order to overcome any obstacles that you find in your way of getting the results you desire and the body you deserve.

- A fitness journal allows you to properly evaluate and document your goals and accomplishments as well as your successes and your failures.

1

- A fitness journal helps you discover how much exercise and how much rest works best for your own particular body type. Every body is different and should be treated as such.

- A fitness journal over time can reveal patterns in your workouts and in your eating habits by keeping track.

- A fitness journal helps you create a workout schedule and regime that is customized to your lifestyle.

- A fitness journal offers you a sense of purpose and accomplishment. It is a great motivator.

- A fitness journal enables you to finally take control and in a sense become your own personal trainer.

- A fitness journal can help you identify concrete goals. It is a great way of recording both short and long term goals as well as tracking your progress in meeting those goals.

- A fitness journal acts as a daily reminder which enables you to become consistent in your workout thereby getting the desired results faster. Consistency in your daily work out can mean the difference between success and failure in meeting the fitness/diet goals that you have set for yourself.

- A fitness journal forces you to remain honest and helps you avoid falling in the pit of useless excuses and lazy procrastination.

How to use this journal?

- This journal can be used as a <u>tool</u> to help you get the most out of your training and fitness regime.

- You can use this journal to <u>set separate goals</u> for yourself in regards to your nutrition, cardiovascular and strength training regime.

- The journal allows you to <u>track short term weekly goals</u> as well as <u>broader long-range goals</u> in the "Overall Goals" section.

- The fitness journal provides space for notes. In the strength training section notes provided you can record details of your strength training regime including; how long you worked out for; which part of your body you excercised; how much weight you lifted; the number of repetitions and sets you did; and the name of the exercise you performed on that given day. There is also space provided so that you can record the distance and duration of your cardio workout. You can also record how you felt in the morning when you first woke up as well as before, during and after each workout. You can record any changes you have noticed in your energy levels, as well as any improvements in your endurance and strength capabilities.

- The fitness journal also provides spaces for notes on Nutrition. In this section you can record and track your eating habits and in time reveal your eating patterns. You can discover which types of foods provide you with the most nutritional value and energy; and what types of foods you should be avoiding for health reasons. You can simply jot down the reasons as to, why you eat when you do, what you eat, how much you routinely eat and how you feel afterward each meal. This is the best way to judge what health plan/diet works best for your own particular body type.

- The fitness journal provides a FAQ section regarding both strength training and nutrition.

- The fitness journal also provides general tips regarding strength training and nutrition in order to help keep you on track in meeting your fitness goals.

Strength Training Section

STRENGTH TRAINING SECTION

- In this section, you can record your strength training exercises, including how much weight you lifted and the number of sets and repetitions you performed.

Example:

EXERCISE	SET1	SET 2	SET3
	REPS/LBS	REPS/LBS	REPS/LBS
Chest press	12/ 80	10/100	8/ 120
Squats	12/75	10/100	8/120
Crunches	60	50	40

Benefits of Strength Training:
- Strength Training helps reduce and even reverse bone loss (potential to reverse the aging process).

- Strength Training provides a number of health benefits and can help reduce the risk of life threatening diseases such as diabetes, heart disease and even cancer. It also aids in preventing osteoporosis.

- Strength Training firms your body. It is the only form of exercise that can reshape your body.

- Strength Training makes you look and feel healthier and more energetic.

- Strength Training helps you lose weight and help keep it off. Exercise boosts one's metabolism and reduces the amount of fat stored in your body which makes it easier to lose weight.

- Strength Training reduces stress and reduces bouts of depression.

- Strength Training has the potential to increase muscle strength and size beyond any other fitness activity.

- Strength Training increases performance in all sports. It can help increase your strength, stamina, and flexibility.

- Strength Training helps to increase your muscle mass. This is essential because muscle burns more calories than fat, so the more muscle mass you have the faster your metabolism.

- Strength Training has important psychological benefits. It gives one a sense of accomplishment after each work out is completed. It improves one's sense of self confidence and body image.

- Strength Training increases brain power by increasing the flow of oxygen to your brain.

FAQ

Should you know the names of each muscle?

- Knowing which exercises target which muscle groups helps you design a more balanced workout program. (See illustration on pg. 8. and pg 9. which points out the major muscles in your body).

Should I use free weights or machines? Try both

- Benefit of Machines-machines support your body and require less coordination than free weights.

- Benefit of Free Weights-free weights force your weaker side to do its share of the work, on a machine your stronger side can take over. You can get faster and better results using free weights. Another benefit to using free weights is that you can do your exercises just about anywhere.

Does the order of my routine matter?

- The basic rule is to work your larger muscle groups before your smaller ones.

How much weight should I lift?

- The amount of weight you should lift depends on your goals; if you want to build the strongest, largest muscles that your body type will allow, lift heavy enough weights so that your muscles tire after 5 or fewer repetitions. If you are seeking moderate results, left weights that cause your muscles to fatigue after 8-15 reps. The last rep that you perform should be the most difficult.

- Gradually increase your weights; your muscles need time to rest.

How long should I rest between sets?

- The heavier your weights, the longer you'll need to rest. Heavy weights = 3 or more minutes, light weights=30 seconds.

How many days a week should I lift weights

- Work each muscle group two or three times a week, and never on consecutive days. Muscles need at least 48 hours to recover from a workout.

How can I avoid getting injured while lifting weights?

- Do a cardiovascular warm-up. (Ex. 5-10 min on the stair climber, rowing machine)

- Use good form-learn the correct posture and technique for each exercise.

- Adjust each machine to fit your body.

- Bend from your knees-not your waist.

- Carry weight plates with two hands and with your elbow bent.

- Ask for someone to "spot" you.

TRAINING TIPS

- Warm-up 5-10 minutes before starting weight training, ie. walking, rowing.

- Exercise the large muscle groups first and work out to the extremities.

- Exhale during the main portion of the exercise and; inhale during the release.

- Use moderate to heavy weights with low reps; rest 2 minutes between each set.

- Do only 2 (maximum 3) exercises per body part. Perform exercises at least 2-3 times per week, per muscle group.

- Periodize-Periodization refers to introducing variety into your workouts by means of reps, sets, rest periods, tempo, intensity, super-sets, eccentric training, etc. The variety is contained in "cycles", usually 1-2 months each. **Why periodize?** Periodization helps to keep your body stimulated and prevent injury while lifting weights.

- Lift Correctly-Make sure the muscles are doing the work by fully contracting each movement. Use full range of motion.

- Cardio must be done-Weight training's main purpose is to strengthen and build lean muscle tissue. In order for weight loss purposes cardiovascular exercise is most effective, it burns calories and fat faster as well as elevating your metabolism. Aim for 3 to 6 days per week of anywhere from 15 to 60 minutes depending on your fitness level and goals.

- Gain Size from Strength-Muscle growth correlates very closely with muscle strength: you don't increase one without increasing the other. To break down muscle tissue, you have to provide a significant amount of stress to the muscle, i.e. heavy weights. Use a weight that keeps you in the range of 4-10 repetitions (lower body and abs no more than 20 reps), depending on what cycle you are in.

- Recuperate-Allow your body and your mind to recover after lifting weights by getting plenty of rest away from the gym and sleeping 7-9 hours each night.

This will keep your body and mind fresh and your energy high. Muscle fibers need 48-72 hours to rebuild. Allow at least 1 day of rest between strength training of the same muscle group.

- Consume Protein-Lifting weights causes you to tear down muscle tissue, which is basically protein. To repair this damage, you'll need more protein. **Sources?** Chicken, egg whites, milk, fish, turkey, tuna, very-lean red meat, and whey protein (powders or in meal replacements).

- Stretching after a muscular exercise program will decrease muscle soreness.

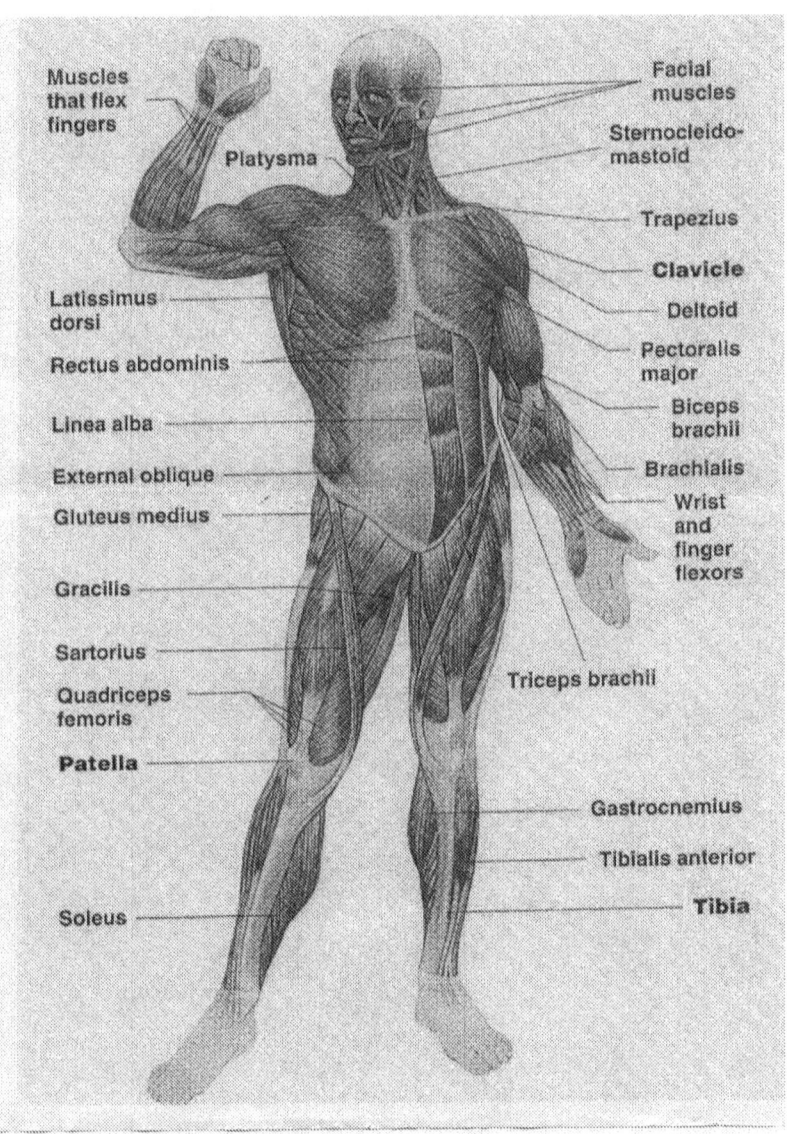

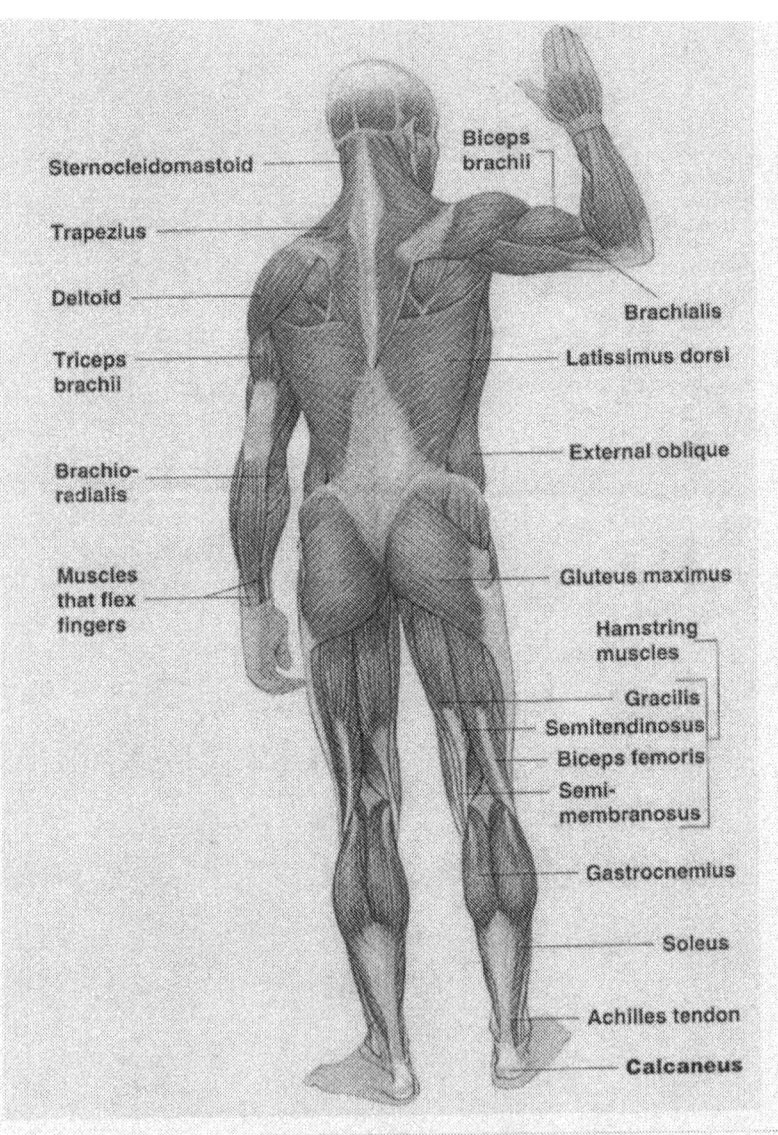

Sternocleidomastoid

Trapezius

Deltoid

Triceps
brachii

Brachio-
radialis

Muscles
that flex
fingers

Biceps
brachii

Brachialis

Latissimus dorsi

External oblique

Gluteus maximus

Hamstring
muscles

Gracilis
Semitendinosus
Biceps femoris
Semi-
membranosus

Gastrocnemius

Soleus

Achilles tendon

Calcaneus

BASIC EXERCISES

LEGS
Squats*
Leg presses
Hack Squats
Lunges
Leg extensions
Calf Raises
Leg curls

CHEST
Bench
Incline/Bench
Deline/Bench
Flys
Dips
Pullovers
Pushups*

BACK
Chin-ups*
Pull-downs
Rows/Seated
Dead Lifts
Row/Bent Over
Hyperextension

SHOULDERS
Presses*
Sidelaterals
Front Raises
Upright Rows
Shrugs
Bent over laterals

TRICEPS
Dips*
Kickbacks
Press downs/Cable
Narrow Grip Bench Press

BICEPS
Curls*
Curls/Reverse
Hammer Curls
Preacher

FOREARMS
Reverse Curls
Wrist Curls

ABDOMINALS
Sit ups
Crunches*
Incline sit-ups
Twisting sit-ups
Leg Raises
Seated Leg Tucks

AEROBICS
Swimming*
Basketball
Walking
Jogging
Biycling
Jump Roping

Recommend

Nutrition Section

Nutrition Section

Nutrition is about why you eat what you eat and how the food you digest affects your body and your health. It is for your best interest health wise to determine which foods and beverages (in which quantities) provide the energy, building material you need to construct and maintain every organ and system in your body. In this section dedicated to nutrition you can track your eating habits daily. You can discover certain patterns over time and find the answers to such questions such as to, why you eat when you eat, and why you make the food choices you do. You can also record such healthy new habits such as replacing bad food choices with healthy substitutes. As you jot down your daily notes you should attempt to be answering these questions?

➢ Did I drink enough water today?

➢ Have I eaten more reduced fat foods?

➢ Have I substituted a fattening food for a more healthier food choice?

➢ Have I attempted to lower my consumption of fried food?

➢ Have I eaten enough fruit and vegetables?

➢ Have I eaten regularly? (ideally every four hours)

➢ Have I chosen my snacks well? (fruits, nuts, hummas, pita bread)

➢ Have I tried to avoid eating food late in the evening?

➢ What were the psychological reasonings behind my food choices?

(For example, do you eat fattening comfort foods when you are feeling depressed?)

Benefits of Balanced nutrition:

- Balanced nutrition in your diet reduces your chances of having high blood pressure, heart disease, a stroke, certain cancers, and the most common kind of diabetes.

- Balanced nutrition contributes to <u>weight loss.</u>

- Balanced nutrition can help <u>reduce stress</u> levels.

- Balanced nutrition can help <u>increase vitality</u> and your body's energy level.

- Balanced nutrition creates a sense of well being.

- Balanced nutrition will build your immune system.

- Balanced nutrition protects cellular integrity and <u>decreases degeneration.</u>

- Balanced nutrition can <u>reduce indigestion</u> discomfort.

- Balanced nutrition can <u>improve fertility.</u>

FAQ

First of all, why should I lose weight?

Your health is the number one reason why you should keep in good shape. If you're more than a few pounds overweight, you increase your risk of getting illnesses and conditions, from heart disease and diabetes to knee and back pain, that will only worsen with age. Getting in shape provides you with a lot more energy, strength and confidence to live the best life you possibly can. It helps you look and feel the best you could.

Why should I lift weights to lose fat?

You may burn more calories in the short-term by doing aerobics than by lifting weights, but it's important to do both, because the more muscle you have, the more calories your body uses in the course of a day (and often those calories will come from your body's fat stores). What's more, a weight-loss program can actually cause you to lose muscle if you don't do anything to stimulate muscle growth.

Why is drinking water so important?

Water reduces fat deposits in the body, flushes out waste and toxins, helps maintain muscle tone, moisturizes skin, and may even suppress appetite. It also carries nutrients, provides joint lubrication and shock absorption, and helps in regulating body temperature. Carry a water bottle with you at all times. Drink water before, during, and after exercise. 8 to 12 glasses each day.

Once I lose the weight can I go back to eating "normally?

A number of people regain weight soon after losing it and often they end up fatter than before. One of the main characteristics of successful fat-losers is consistency: No matter what program you're on, it won't work unless you stay with it. After you have reached your target weight you should enter a maintenance program which means sticking to an overall healthy new approach to eating and exercising. At that stage, it's okay to cheat a little here and there, as long as you stick to your nutrition and training regimens.

FAQ (CON'T)

How healthy are "nonfat" or "low-fat" foods?

Advertising a food as "fat-free," "low-fat" or "reduced fat" is a pervasive marketing gimmick, but does not necessarily mean the food is good for you. In snack foods, the fat is often replaced by copious amounts of sugar or refined flour that has little nutritional value and easily translates to fat, so you shouldn't be eating these anyway. But you should look for reduced-fat meat and milk products, which are usually lower in calories and higher in protein than their full-fat versions. Here is what the labels mean:

➤ *Fat-free* refers to anything that has less than half a gram of fat per serving. (Make sure you know how big-or small-a serving is.)

➤ *Low-fat* means the product has fewer than three grams of fat per serving.

➤ Reduced fat is a label often seen on junk foods such as ice cream and candy bars, and merely means that the product has at least 25 percent less fat than the regular version.

➤ *Lean* is a label you'll sometimes find on meat and poultry. It means there's less than 10g of fat (and less than 4.5g of saturated fat) per 100 grams (3.5 ounces).

➤ *Extra* lean has less than 5g of fat and less than 2g saturated fat per 100 grams.

Note: If you cannot avoid diet foods, at least stick with the fat-free versions (but remember, they'll likely be packed with some form of sugar).

Are all carbs, protein and fat the same?

You need to choose the kinds of foods you eat carefully, because this helps determine both how much you can eat without going hungry and how many calories you'll burn.

➤ *Carbohydrates* Ease up on dry, refined carbs (such as white bread, crackers or cookies), which provide calories without satisfying hunger very well, causing you to eat too much too quickly. Instead, focus on "wet," fiber-rich carbs such as fruits, vegetables, cooked brown rice and baked potatoes, which provide plenty of bulk so you eat less. Just as important, avoid drinking your carbs in the form of soda or beer, since liquid does almost nothing to stop the munchies.

➤ *Fats* have more than twice the calories by weight than carbs or protein, but you still need some in your diet to stay healthy and avoid those hunger pangs. The ones to cut way down on are saturated fats (coconut oil, palm kernel oil, butter, beef fat, lard and dairy fat) and hydrogenated fats, also called trans-fatty acids (vegetable shortenings and margarine, often found in snack foods). Instead, add a few nuts, a little olive oil and especially fish to your meals. The omega-3 fatty acids in these foods are much more healthful than other fats; what's more, they may also aid in weight loss by slowing down a fat-forming enzyme in your body.

➤ *Protein* will help keep your blood-sugar levels steady and curb your appetite, perhaps even raising your body temperature so you burn more calories. But many foods rich in protein are also high in saturated fat, so choose fat-free dairy products, lean cuts of meat and poultry, all kinds of fish, and vegetarian protein sources such as beans and soy.

THE FOOD GUIDE PYRAMID

The Food Guide Pyramid is an outline of what to eat each day. It's not a rigid prescription but a general guide that lets you choose a healthful diet that's right for you. The Pyramid calls for eating a variety of foods to get the nutrients you need and at the same time the right amount of calories to maintain healthy weight. Start with plenty of breads, cereals, rice, pasta, vegetables, and fruits. Add 2-3 servings from the milk group and 2-3 servings from the meat group. Remember to go easy on fats, oils, and sweets, the foods in the small tip of the Pyramid.

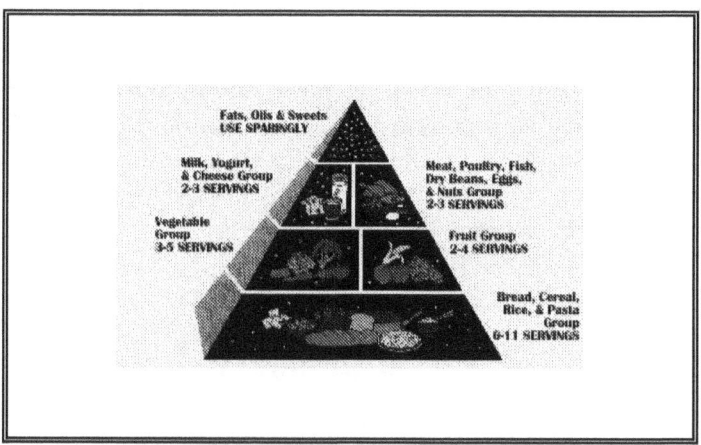

Nutritional Sources and Information

BASIC NUTRITIONAL BALANCE

1. Protein   12%
2. Carbohydrates   58%
3. Fat   30%
4. Vitamins
5. Minerals
6. Water

PROTEIN

Egg Whites	Whole Grain Wheat
Fish	Cheese
Cows Milk	Soy Beans
Lean Beef	Chicken/Turkey

FATS

Eggs	Dairy Products
Red Meat	Oils

CARBOHYDRATES (simple)

Fruit*

CARBOHYDRATES (complex)

Potatoes	Vegetables
Rice	
Pasta	
Bread	

EMPTY CALORIES (limit intake)

Cake
Soft Drinks
Candy
Processed foods with sugar

Nutrition/Diet Tips

- To lose body fat you must eat fewer calories than your body burns off, so EAT LESS—but you must NOT starve yourself, otherwise you will lose more muscle than fat!

- Start eating 5-6 meals per day (space them out to about one every 3 hours). You are eating more often, but not necessarily more. Research shows that eating more frequently, with each meal consisting of both protein and carbohydrates, will provide you with the following benefits:

  ➢ Increased nutrient absorption

  ➢ Stabilized energy levels

  ➢ Increased muscle growth

  ➢ Decreased indigestion

  ➢ Controlled appetite

- Balance the food you eat with physical activity in order to maintain or improve your weight. Exercise increases muscles, and reduces the amount of fat stored in your body.

- Increase your protein intake. Without protein your body cannot build new muscle. Protein also helps to increase your metabolism—which burns calories.

- Drink tons of water.

- Get rid of junk food. (provides few nutrients and lots of empty calories") Examples include cookies, pastries, candy and processed goods.

- Eat a variety of foods to ensure you are maintaining the amount of proper nutrients your body need.

- Keep healthy snacks handy; such as celery, carrots, protein bars, etc.

- Have a shake. Ready-to-drink meals and meal replacement powders, when combined with your regular diet, help keep fat intake down and offer a lot of convenience.

- Don't skip meals. Starving yourself only lowers your bodies metabolism (it tries to hold on to everything it has) and creates uneven energy levels throughout the day making you very hungry. Sooner or later, you'll give in and over consume. Skipping meals also makes it hard to exercise because you'll have less energy.

- Alcohol facts. Alcohol is the only form of calorie your muscles CANNOT burn for fuel. Alcohol slows your metabolism. Alcohol also stimulates your appetite for fatty foods.

Nutrition/Diet Tips

- Eat breakfast. This should be the largest meal of the day, yet people often skip it completely. Eating breakfast gives you a head start on an energized and healthy day. Also, not eating breakfast may cause your resting metabolic rate to dip by 5 percent-a small decline that may creep up to a 10-pound weight gain in a year's time.

- Don't eat 2 hours before bed. Don't consume any carbohydrates within 3 hours before bed, or it will be stored as body fat.

- Read the labels. The FDA has done a great job making information available to consumers.

- "Treat" yourself. Reward yourself one day a week by eating something like ice cream, cheeseburger, pizza or whatever you know is a "forbidden" food. But do this ONLY if you've been good!

- Choose a diet that includes plenty of grain products as well as fruits and vegetables. It is recommended to have 2-3 servings of fruits and 3-5 servings of vegetables each day.

- Chose a diet low in fat, saturated fat, and cholesterol. Limit: chocolate, alcohol, hard candy, cake, cookies, pie, frozen yogurt, non-diet soft drinks, pancake syrup, jams, brown sugar, and raw sugar.

WHAT BODYFAT CATEGORY ARE YOU IN?

Classification	Women (%fat)	Men (%fat)
Essential Fat	10-12%	2-4%
Athletes	14-20%	6-13%
General Fitness	21-24%	14-17%
Acceptable	25-31%	18-25%
Obese	32% and higher	25% and higher
Source: American Council on Exercise		

TRACKING YOUR PERSONAL GOALS!

To obtain the strongest, healthiest and sexist body that you can possibly possess, you will have to **<u>EARN</u>** it.

E-EXERCISE (WEIGHT TRAINING)
A-AREOBIC (CARDIO 3-4 DAYS PER WEEK)
R-REST (SLEEP 7-8 HOURS DAY, MININUM)
N-NURTITION (EATING HEALTHIER)

Good luck on your voyage to obtain a healthier and more satisfying life!

*Overall goals:

_____

_____

_____

_____

_____

_____

_____

_____

_____

*Cardio exercise goals:

_____

_____

_____

_____

_____

_____

_____

_____

_____

*Strength-training goals:

_____
_____
_____
_____
_____
_____
_____
_____
_____

*Nutrition goals:

_____
_____
_____
_____
_____
_____
_____
_____
_____

DATE:

_____

BREAKFAST:

At: _____

LUNCH:

At: _____

DINNER:

At: _____

SNACKS:

At: _____

At: _____

At: _____

At: _____

NOTES:

_____

_____

_____

_____

_____

WEIGHT: _____ *LBS*
           _____ *AM/PM*

DATE _____   TIME _____   BODY AREA _____

EXERCISE	SET 1 REPS/LBS	SET 2 REPS/LBS	SET 3 REPS/LBS	SET 4 REPS/LBS	SET 5 REPS/LBS	SET 6 REPS/LBS

CARDIO EXERCISE:

_____

_____

_____

_____

NOTES:

_____

_____

_____

_____

DATE:

_____

BREAKFAST:

At: _____

LUNCH:

At: _____

DINNER:

At: _____

SNACKS:
At: _____

At: _____

At: _____

At: _____

NOTES:

_____

_____

_____

_____

_____

WEIGHT: _____ *LBS*
              _____ *AM/PM*

DATE _____ TIME _____ BODY AREA _____

EXERCISE	SET 1 REPS/LBS	SET 2 REPS/LBS	SET 3 REPS/LBS	SET 4 REPS/LBS	SET 5 REPS/LBS	SET 6 REPS/LBS

CARDIO EXERCISE:

_____

_____

_____

_____

NOTES:

_____

_____

_____

_____

DATE:

_____

BREAKFAST:
_____
At: _____
_____

LUNCH:
_____
At: _____
_____

DINNER:
_____
At: _____
_____

SNACKS:
At: _____
_____
At: _____
_____
At: _____
_____
At: _____
_____

NOTES:
_____
_____
_____
_____
_____

WEIGHT: _____ *LBS*
                 _____ *AM/PM*

DATE _____

TIME _____

BODY AREA _____

EXERCISE	SET 1 REPS/LBS	SET 2 REPS/LBS	SET 3 REPS/LBS	SET 4 REPS/LBS	SET 5 REPS/LBS	SET 6 REPS/LBS

CARDIO EXERCISE:

_____

_____

_____

_____

NOTES:

_____

_____

_____

_____

DATE: _____

BREAKFAST:

_____
At: _____
_____

LUNCH:

_____
At: _____
_____

DINNER:

_____
At: _____
_____

SNACKS:
At: _____
_____
At: _____
_____
At: _____
_____
At: _____
_____

NOTES:

_____
_____
_____
_____
_____

WEIGHT: _____ *LBS*
                 _____ *AM/PM*

DATE   **TIME**   **BODY AREA**

_____   _____   _____

| EXERCISE | SET 1 | SET 2 | SET 3 | SET 4 | SET 5 | SET 6 |
	REPS/LBS	REPS/LBS	REPS/LBS	REPS/LBS	REPS/LBS	REPS/LBS

CARDIO EXERCISE:

_____

_____

_____

_____

NOTES:

_____

_____

_____

_____

DATE:

_____

BREAKFAST:

_____

At: _____

LUNCH:

_____

At: _____

DINNER:

_____

At: _____

SNACKS:
At: _____

At: _____

At: _____

At: _____

NOTES:

_____

_____

_____

_____

_____

WEIGHT: _____ *LBS*
                 _____ *AM/PM*

DATE   **TIME**   **BODY AREA**

EXERCISE	SET 1	SET 2	SET 3	SET 4	SET 5	SET 6
	REPS/LBS	REPS/LBS	REPS/LBS	REPS/LBS	REPS/LBS	REPS/LBS

CARDIO EXERCISE:

_____

_____

_____

_____

NOTES:

_____

_____

_____

_____

DATE: _____

BREAKFAST:

At: _____ _____

LUNCH:

At: _____ _____

DINNER:

At: _____ _____

SNACKS:

At: _____ _____

At: _____ _____

At: _____ _____

At: _____ _____

NOTES:

_____

_____

_____

_____

_____

WEIGHT: _____ *LBS*

_____ *AM/PM*

DATE _____

TIME _____

BODY AREA _____

EXERCISE	SET 1	SET 2	SET 3	SET 4	SET 5	SET 6
	REPS/LBS	REPS/LBS	REPS/LBS	REPS/LBS	REPS/LBS	REPS/LBS

CARDIO EXERCISE:

_____

_____

_____

_____

NOTES:

_____

_____

_____

_____

DATE:
_____

BREAKFAST:

At: _____ _____

_____

LUNCH:

At: _____ _____

_____

DINNER:

At: _____ _____

_____

SNACKS:

At: _____ _____

At: _____ _____

At: _____ _____

At: _____ _____

NOTES:

_____

_____

_____

_____

_____

WEIGHT: _____ *LBS*

             _____ *AM/PM*

DATE
_____

TIME
_____

BODY AREA
_____

EXERCISE	SET 1	SET 2	SET 3	SET 4	SET 5	SET 6
	REPS/LBS	REPS/LBS	REPS/LBS	REPS/LBS	REPS/LBS	REPS/LBS

CARDIO EXERCISE:

_____
_____
_____
_____

NOTES:

_____
_____
_____
_____

DATE:

_____

BREAKFAST:
_____
At: _____
_____

LUNCH:
_____
At: _____
_____

DINNER:
_____
At: _____
_____

SNACKS:
At: _____
_____
At: _____
_____
At: _____
_____
At: _____
_____

NOTES:
_____
_____
_____
_____
_____

WEIGHT: _____ *LBS*
              _____ *AM/PM*

DATE   **TIME**   **BODY AREA**

EXERCISE	SET 1	SET 2	SET 3	SET 4	SET 5	SET 6
	REPS/LBS	REPS/LBS	REPS/LBS	REPS/LBS	REPS/LBS	REPS/LBS

CARDIO EXERCISE:

_____

_____

_____

_____

NOTES:

_____

_____

_____

_____

DATE:

_____

BREAKFAST:

_____

At: _____

_____

LUNCH:

_____

At: _____

_____

DINNER:

_____

At: _____

_____

SNACKS:

At: _____

_____

At: _____

_____

At: _____

_____

At: _____

_____

NOTES:

_____

_____

_____

_____

_____

WEIGHT: _____ *LBS*

              _____ *AM/PM*

DATE   **TIME**   **BODY AREA**

_____   _____   _____

EXERCISE	SET 1	SET 2	SET 3	SET 4	SET 5	SET 6
	REPS/LBS	REPS/LBS	REPS/LBS	REPS/LBS	REPS/LBS	REPS/LBS

CARDIO EXERCISE:

_____

_____

_____

_____

NOTES:

_____

_____

_____

_____

DATE:

_____

BREAKFAST:

At: _____

LUNCH:

At: _____

DINNER:

At: _____

SNACKS:
At: _____

At: _____

At: _____

At: _____

NOTES:

_____

_____

_____

_____

_____

WEIGHT: _____ **LBS**
                 _____ **AM/PM**

DATE _____   TIME _____   BODY AREA _____

EXERCISE	SET 1	SET 2	SET 3	SET 4	SET 5	SET 6
	REPS/LBS	REPS/LBS	REPS/LBS	REPS/LBS	REPS/LBS	REPS/LBS

CARDIO EXERCISE:

_____

_____

_____

_____

NOTES:

_____

_____

_____

_____

DATE:

BREAKFAST:

At: _____

LUNCH:

At: _____

DINNER:

At: _____

SNACKS:
At: _____

At: _____

At: _____

At: _____

NOTES:

WEIGHT: _____ *LBS*
              _____ *AM/PM*

DATE   **TIME**   **BODY AREA**

EXERCISE	SET 1	SET 2	SET 3	SET 4	SET 5	SET 6
	REPS/LBS	REPS/LBS	REPS/LBS	REPS/LBS	REPS/LBS	REPS/LBS

CARDIO EXERCISE:

_____

_____

_____

_____

NOTES:

_____

_____

_____

_____

DATE:

_____

BREAKFAST:

At: _____
_____

LUNCH:

At: _____
_____

DINNER:

At: _____
_____

SNACKS:
At: _____
_____

At: _____
_____

At: _____
_____

At: _____
_____

NOTES:

_____

_____

_____

_____

_____

WEIGHT: _____ *LBS*
                 _____ *AM/PM*

DATE   TIME   BODY AREA

_____   _____   _____

EXERCISE	SET 1	SET 2	SET 3	SET 4	SET 5	SET 6
	REPS/LBS	REPS/LBS	REPS/LBS	REPS/LBS	REPS/LBS	REPS/LBS

CARDIO EXERCISE:

_____

_____

_____

_____

NOTES:

_____

_____

_____

_____

DATE:
_____

BREAKFAST:

At: _____
_____

LUNCH:

At: _____
_____

DINNER:

At: _____
_____

SNACKS:
At: _____
_____

At: _____
_____

At: _____
_____

At: _____
_____

NOTES:

_____

_____

_____

_____

_____

WEIGHT:　_____ *LBS*
　　　　　　 _____ *AM/PM*

DATE

TIME

BODY AREA

EXERCISE	SET 1	SET 2	SET 3	SET 4	SET 5	SET 6
	REPS/LBS	REPS/LBS	REPS/LBS	REPS/LBS	REPS/LBS	REPS/LBS

CARDIO EXERCISE:

_____

_____

_____

_____

NOTES:

_____

_____

_____

_____

DATE:

BREAKFAST:

At: _____

LUNCH:

At: _____

DINNER:

At: _____

SNACKS:
At: _____

At: _____

At: _____

At: _____

NOTES:

WEIGHT: _____ *LBS*
              _____ *AM/PM*

DATE   TIME   BODY AREA

_____   _____   _____

EXERCISE	SET 1	SET 2	SET 3	SET 4	SET 5	SET 6
	REPS/LBS	REPS/LBS	REPS/LBS	REPS/LBS	REPS/LBS	REPS/LBS

CARDIO EXERCISE:

_____

_____

_____

_____

NOTES:

_____

_____

_____

_____

DATE:
_____

BREAKFAST:

At: _____
_____

LUNCH:

At: _____
_____

DINNER:

At: _____
_____

SNACKS:
At: _____
_____

At: _____
_____

At: _____
_____

At: _____
_____

NOTES:

_____

_____

_____

_____

_____

WEIGHT: _____ *LBS*
                 _____ *AM/PM*

DATE   TIME   BODY AREA

_____   _____   _____

EXERCISE	SET 1	SET 2	SET 3	SET 4	SET 5	SET 6
	REPS/LBS	REPS/LBS	REPS/LBS	REPS/LBS	REPS/LBS	REPS/LBS

CARDIO EXERCISE:

_____

_____

_____

_____

NOTES:

_____

_____

_____

_____

DATE:

_____

BREAKFAST:

_____

At: _____

_____

LUNCH:

_____

At: _____

_____

DINNER:

_____

At: _____

_____

SNACKS:

At: _____

_____

At: _____

_____

At: _____

_____

At: _____

_____

NOTES:

_____

_____

_____

_____

_____

WEIGHT: _____ *LBS*

                 _____ *AM/PM*

DATE   TIME   BODY AREA

EXERCISE	SET 1	SET 2	SET 3	SET 4	SET 5	SET 6
	REPS/LBS	REPS/LBS	REPS/LBS	REPS/LBS	REPS/LBS	REPS/LBS

CARDIO EXERCISE:

_____

_____

_____

_____

NOTES:

_____

_____

_____

_____

DATE:

_____

BREAKFAST:

_____
At: _____
_____

LUNCH:

_____
At: _____
_____

DINNER:

_____
At: _____
_____

SNACKS:
At: _____
_____
At: _____
_____
At: _____
_____
At: _____
_____

NOTES:

_____

_____

_____

_____

_____

WEIGHT:　　_____ *LBS*
　　　　　　　_____ *AM/PM*

DATE   **TIME**   **BODY AREA**

_____   _____   _____

EXERCISE	SET 1	SET 2	SET 3	SET 4	SET 5	SET 6
	REPS/LBS	REPS/LBS	REPS/LBS	REPS/LBS	REPS/LBS	REPS/LBS

CARDIO EXERCISE:

_____

_____

_____

_____

NOTES:

_____

_____

_____

_____

DATE:
_____

BREAKFAST:
_____
At: _____
_____

LUNCH:
_____
At: _____
_____

DINNER:
_____
At: _____
_____

SNACKS:
At: _____
_____
At: _____
_____
At: _____
_____
At: _____
_____

NOTES:

_____

_____

_____

_____

_____

WEIGHT: _____ *LBS*
                 _____ *AM/PM*

DATE   **TIME**   **BODY AREA**

_____   _____   _____

EXERCISE	SET 1	SET 2	SET 3	SET 4	SET 5	SET 6
	REPS/LBS	REPS/LBS	REPS/LBS	REPS/LBS	REPS/LBS	REPS/LBS

CARDIO EXERCISE:

_____

_____

_____

_____

NOTES:

_____

_____

_____

_____

DATE: _____

BREAKFAST:
_____
At: _____
_____

LUNCH:
_____
At: _____
_____

DINNER:
_____
At: _____
_____

SNACKS:
At: _____
_____
At: _____
_____
At: _____
_____
At: _____
_____

NOTES:

_____
_____
_____
_____
_____

WEIGHT: _____ *LBS*
_____ *AM/PM*

DATE   TIME   BODY AREA

_____   _____   _____

EXERCISE	SET 1 REPS/LBS	SET 2 REPS/LBS	SET 3 REPS/LBS	SET 4 REPS/LBS	SET 5 REPS/LBS	SET 6 REPS/LBS

CARDIO EXERCISE:

_____

_____

_____

_____

NOTES:

_____

_____

_____

_____

DATE:

BREAKFAST:

At: _____

LUNCH:

At: _____

DINNER:

At: _____

SNACKS:

At: _____

At: _____

At: _____

At: _____

NOTES:

WEIGHT: _____ **LBS**
_____ **AM/PM**

DATE

TIME

BODY AREA

_____

_____

_____

EXERCISE	SET 1	SET 2	SET 3	SET 4	SET 5	SET 6
	REPS/LBS	REPS/LBS	REPS/LBS	REPS/LBS	REPS/LBS	REPS/LBS

CARDIO EXERCISE:

_____

_____

_____

_____

NOTES:

_____

_____

_____

_____

DATE:

_____

BREAKFAST:

At: _____

LUNCH:

At: _____

DINNER:

At: _____

SNACKS:
At: _____

At: _____

At: _____

At: _____

NOTES:

_____

_____

_____

_____

_____

WEIGHT: _____ *LBS*
              _____ *AM/PM*

DATE

TIME

BODY AREA

_____   _____   _____

EXERCISE	SET 1	SET 2	SET 3	SET 4	SET 5	SET 6
	REPS/LBS	REPS/LBS	REPS/LBS	REPS/LBS	REPS/LBS	REPS/LBS

CARDIO EXERCISE:

_____

_____

_____

_____

NOTES:

_____

_____

_____

_____

DATE:
_____

BREAKFAST:

At: _____
_____

LUNCH:

At: _____
_____

DINNER:

At: _____
_____

SNACKS:
At: _____

At: _____
_____

At: _____
_____

At: _____
_____

NOTES:

_____

_____

_____

_____

_____

WEIGHT: _____ *LBS*
              _____ *AM/PM*

DATE

TIME

BODY AREA

_____

EXERCISE	SET 1	SET 2	SET 3	SET 4	SET 5	SET 6
	REPS/LBS	REPS/LBS	REPS/LBS	REPS/LBS	REPS/LBS	REPS/LBS

CARDIO EXERCISE:

_____

_____

_____

_____

NOTES:

_____

_____

_____

_____

DATE:
_____

BREAKFAST:

At: _____
_____

LUNCH:

At: _____
_____

DINNER:

At: _____
_____

SNACKS:
At: _____

At: _____
_____

At: _____
_____

At: _____
_____

NOTES:

_____

_____

_____

_____

_____

WEIGHT: _____ *LBS*
                 _____ *AM/PM*

DATE   TIME   BODY AREA

_____   _____   _____

EXERCISE	SET 1	SET 2	SET 3	SET 4	SET 5	SET 6
	REPS/LBS	REPS/LBS	REPS/LBS	REPS/LBS	REPS/LBS	REPS/LBS

CARDIO EXERCISE:

_____

_____

_____

_____

NOTES:

_____

_____

_____

_____

DATE:

BREAKFAST:

At: _____

LUNCH:

At: _____

DINNER:

At: _____

SNACKS:
At: _____

At: _____

At: _____

At: _____

NOTES:

WEIGHT: _____ *LBS*
_____ *AM/PM*

DATE _____   **TIME** _____   **BODY AREA** _____

EXERCISE	SET 1 REPS/LBS	SET 2 REPS/LBS	SET 3 REPS/LBS	SET 4 REPS/LBS	SET 5 REPS/LBS	SET 6 REPS/LBS

CARDIO EXERCISE:

_____

_____

_____

_____

NOTES:

_____

_____

_____

_____

DATE:
_____

BREAKFAST:

At: _____ _____

_____

LUNCH:

At: _____ _____

_____

DINNER:

At: _____ _____

_____

SNACKS:

At: _____ _____

At: _____ _____

At: _____ _____

At: _____ _____

NOTES:

_____

_____

_____

_____

_____

WEIGHT: _____ *LBS*

_____ *AM/PM*

DATE

TIME

BODY AREA

EXERCISE	SET 1 REPS/LBS	SET 2 REPS/LBS	SET 3 REPS/LBS	SET 4 REPS/LBS	SET 5 REPS/LBS	SET 6 REPS/LBS

CARDIO EXERCISE:

_____

_____

_____

_____

NOTES:

_____

_____

_____

_____

DATE:

BREAKFAST:

At: _____

LUNCH:

At: _____

DINNER:

At: _____

SNACKS:
At: _____

At: _____

At: _____

At: _____

NOTES:

WEIGHT: _____ *LBS*
_____ *AM/PM*

DATE   TIME   BODY AREA

_____   _____   _____

EXERCISE	SET 1	SET 2	SET 3	SET 4	SET 5	SET 6
	REPS/LBS	REPS/LBS	REPS/LBS	REPS/LBS	REPS/LBS	REPS/LBS

CARDIO EXERCISE:

_____

_____

_____

_____

NOTES:

_____

_____

_____

_____

DATE:

_____

BREAKFAST:

At: _____

LUNCH:

At: _____

DINNER:

At: _____

SNACKS:

At: _____

At: _____

At: _____

At: _____

NOTES:

_____

_____

_____

_____

_____

WEIGHT: _____ *LBS*

              _____ *AM/PM*

DATE   **TIME**   **BODY AREA**

_____   _____   _____

EXERCISE	SET 1	SET 2	SET 3	SET 4	SET 5	SET 6
	REPS/LBS	REPS/LBS	REPS/LBS	REPS/LBS	REPS/LBS	REPS/LBS

CARDIO EXERCISE:

_____

_____

_____

_____

NOTES:

_____

_____

_____

_____

DATE:
_____

BREAKFAST:
_____
At: _____
_____

LUNCH:
_____
At: _____
_____

DINNER:
_____
At: _____
_____

SNACKS:
At: _____
_____
At: _____
_____
At: _____
_____
At: _____
_____

NOTES:
_____
_____
_____
_____
_____

WEIGHT: _____ **LBS**
                 _____ **AM/PM**

DATE   TIME   BODY AREA

_____   _____   _____

EXERCISE	SET 1	SET 2	SET 3	SET 4	SET 5	SET 6
	REPS/LBS	REPS/LBS	REPS/LBS	REPS/LBS	REPS/LBS	REPS/LBS

CARDIO EXERCISE:

_____

_____

_____

_____

NOTES:

_____

_____

_____

_____

DATE:
_____

BREAKFAST:

At: _____ _____

_____

LUNCH:

At: _____ _____

_____

DINNER:

At: _____ _____

_____

SNACKS:
At: _____ _____

At: _____ _____

At: _____ _____

At: _____ _____

NOTES:

_____

_____

_____

_____

_____

WEIGHT: _____ *LBS*
                 _____ *AM/PM*

DATE _____   **TIME** _____   **BODY AREA** _____

EXERCISE	SET 1	SET 2	SET 3	SET 4	SET 5	SET 6
	REPS/LBS	REPS/LBS	REPS/LBS	REPS/LBS	REPS/LBS	REPS/LBS

CARDIO EXERCISE:

_____

_____

_____

_____

NOTES:

_____

_____

_____

_____

DATE:
_____

BREAKFAST:
_____
At: _____
_____

LUNCH:
_____
At: _____
_____

DINNER:
_____
At: _____
_____

SNACKS:
At: _____
_____
At: _____
_____
At: _____
_____
At: _____
_____

NOTES:

_____
_____
_____
_____
_____

WEIGHT: _____ *LBS*
               _____ *AM/PM*

DATE _____   TIME _____   BODY AREA _____

EXERCISE	SET 1 REPS/LBS	SET 2 REPS/LBS	SET 3 REPS/LBS	SET 4 REPS/LBS	SET 5 REPS/LBS	SET 6 REPS/LBS

CARDIO EXERCISE:

_____

_____

_____

_____

NOTES:

_____

_____

_____

_____

DATE:
_____

BREAKFAST:
_____
At: _____
_____

LUNCH:
_____
At: _____
_____

DINNER:
_____
At: _____
_____

SNACKS:
At: _____
_____
At: _____
_____
At: _____
_____
At: _____
_____

NOTES:

_____
_____
_____
_____
_____

WEIGHT: _____ *LBS*
                _____ *AM/PM*

DATE   **TIME**   **BODY AREA**

_____   _____   _____

EXERCISE	SET 1	SET 2	SET 3	SET 4	SET 5	SET 6
	REPS/LBS	REPS/LBS	REPS/LBS	REPS/LBS	REPS/LBS	REPS/LBS

CARDIO EXERCISE:

_____

_____

_____

_____

NOTES:

_____

_____

_____

_____

DATE:

_____

BREAKFAST:
_____
At: _____
_____

LUNCH:
_____
At: _____
_____

DINNER:
_____
At: _____
_____

SNACKS:
At: _____
_____
At: _____
_____
At: _____
_____
At: _____
_____

NOTES:

_____

_____

_____

_____

_____

WEIGHT: _____ *LBS*
                 _____ *AM/PM*

DATE   **TIME**   **BODY AREA**

_____   _____   _____

EXERCISE	SET 1	SET 2	SET 3	SET 4	SET 5	SET 6
	REPS/LBS	REPS/LBS	REPS/LBS	REPS/LBS	REPS/LBS	REPS/LBS

CARDIO EXERCISE:

_____

_____

_____

_____

NOTES:

_____

_____

_____

_____

DATE:
_____

BREAKFAST:

At: _____
_____

LUNCH:

At: _____
_____

DINNER:

At: _____
_____

SNACKS:
At: _____

At: _____

At: _____

At: _____

NOTES:

_____

_____

_____

_____

_____

WEIGHT: _____ LBS
           _____ AM/PM

DATE   TIME   BODY AREA

_____   _____   _____

EXERCISE	SET 1	SET 2	SET 3	SET 4	SET 5	SET 6
	REPS/LBS	REPS/LBS	REPS/LBS	REPS/LBS	REPS/LBS	REPS/LBS

CARDIO EXERCISE:

_____

_____

_____

_____

NOTES:

_____

_____

_____

_____

DATE:

_____

BREAKFAST:

At: _____

LUNCH:

At: _____

DINNER:

At: _____

SNACKS:
At: _____

At: _____

At: _____

At: _____

NOTES:

_____

_____

_____

_____

_____

WEIGHT: _____ *LBS*
          _____ *AM/PM*

DATE   TIME   BODY AREA

_____   _____   _____

EXERCISE	SET 1	SET 2	SET 3	SET 4	SET 5	SET 6
	REPS/LBS	REPS/LBS	REPS/LBS	REPS/LBS	REPS/LBS	REPS/LBS

CARDIO EXERCISE:

_____

_____

_____

_____

NOTES:

_____

_____

_____

_____

DATE:

_____

BREAKFAST:

_____

At: _____

_____

LUNCH:

_____

At: _____

_____

DINNER:

_____

At: _____

_____

SNACKS:
At: _____

_____

At: _____

_____

At: _____

_____

At: _____

_____

NOTES:

_____

_____

_____

_____

_____

WEIGHT: _____ *LBS*
              _____ *AM/PM*

DATE **TIME** **BODY AREA**

_____ _____ _____

EXERCISE	SET 1	SET 2	SET 3	SET 4	SET 5	SET 6
	REPS/LBS	REPS/LBS	REPS/LBS	REPS/LBS	REPS/LBS	REPS/LBS

CARDIO EXERCISE:

_____

_____

_____

_____

NOTES:

_____

_____

_____

_____

DATE:

_____

BREAKFAST:

At: _____

LUNCH:

At: _____

DINNER:

At: _____

SNACKS:
At: _____

At: _____

At: _____

At: _____

NOTES:

_____

_____

_____

_____

_____

WEIGHT: _____ *LBS*

_____ *AM/PM*

DATE   TIME   BODY AREA

EXERCISE	SET 1	SET 2	SET 3	SET 4	SET 5	SET 6
	REPS/LBS	REPS/LBS	REPS/LBS	REPS/LBS	REPS/LBS	REPS/LBS

CARDIO EXERCISE:

_____
_____
_____
_____

NOTES:

_____
_____
_____
_____

DATE:

_____

BREAKFAST:

At: _____

LUNCH:

At: _____

DINNER:

At: _____

SNACKS:

At: _____

At: _____

At: _____

At: _____

NOTES:

_____

_____

_____

_____

_____

WEIGHT: _____ **LBS**

               _____ **AM/PM**

DATE   TIME   BODY AREA

_____   _____   _____

EXERCISE	SET 1	SET 2	SET 3	SET 4	SET 5	SET 6
	REPS/LBS	REPS/LBS	REPS/LBS	REPS/LBS	REPS/LBS	REPS/LBS

CARDIO EXERCISE:

_____

_____

_____

_____

NOTES:

_____

_____

_____

_____

DATE:

_____

BREAKFAST:

_____

At: _____

LUNCH:

_____

At: _____

DINNER:

_____

At: _____

SNACKS:
At: _____

_____

At: _____

_____

At: _____

_____

At: _____

NOTES:

_____

_____

_____

_____

_____

WEIGHT: _____ *LBS*
                 _____ *AM/PM*

DATE   TIME   BODY AREA

_____   _____   _____

EXERCISE	SET 1	SET 2	SET 3	SET 4	SET 5	SET 6
	REPS/LBS	REPS/LBS	REPS/LBS	REPS/LBS	REPS/LBS	REPS/LBS

CARDIO EXERCISE:

_____

_____

_____

_____

NOTES:

_____

_____

_____

_____

DATE:

_____

BREAKFAST:

At: _____

_____

LUNCH:

At: _____

_____

DINNER:

At: _____

_____

SNACKS:
At: _____

At: _____

At: _____

At: _____

NOTES:

_____

_____

_____

_____

_____

WEIGHT: _____ *LBS*
            _____ *AM/PM*

DATE _____ TIME _____ BODY AREA _____

EXERCISE	SET 1 REPS/LBS	SET 2 REPS/LBS	SET 3 REPS/LBS	SET 4 REPS/LBS	SET 5 REPS/LBS	SET 6 REPS/LBS

CARDIO EXERCISE:

_____
_____
_____
_____

NOTES:

_____
_____
_____
_____

DATE:

_____

BREAKFAST:

_____

At: _____

_____

LUNCH:

_____

At: _____

_____

DINNER:

_____

At: _____

_____

SNACKS:
At: _____

_____

At: _____

_____

At: _____

_____

At: _____

_____

NOTES:

_____

_____

_____

_____

_____

WEIGHT: _____ *LBS*
                 _____ *AM/PM*

DATE

TIME

BODY AREA

_____

_____

_____

EXERCISE	SET 1 REPS/LBS	SET 2 REPS/LBS	SET 3 REPS/LBS	SET 4 REPS/LBS	SET 5 REPS/LBS	SET 6 REPS/LBS

CARDIO EXERCISE:

_____

_____

_____

_____

NOTES:

_____

_____

_____

_____

DATE:

BREAKFAST:

At: _____

LUNCH:

At: _____

DINNER:

At: _____

SNACKS:
At: _____

At: _____

At: _____

At: _____

NOTES:

WEIGHT: _____ *LBS*

_____ *AM/PM*

DATE   **TIME**   **BODY AREA**

_____   _____   _____

EXERCISE	SET 1 REPS/LBS	SET 2 REPS/LBS	SET 3 REPS/LBS	SET 4 REPS/LBS	SET 5 REPS/LBS	SET 6 REPS/LBS

CARDIO EXERCISE:

_____

_____

_____

_____

NOTES:

_____

_____

_____

_____

DATE:
_____

BREAKFAST:
_____
At: _____
_____

LUNCH:
_____
At: _____
_____

DINNER:
_____
At: _____
_____

SNACKS:
At: _____
_____
At: _____
_____
At: _____
_____
At: _____
_____

NOTES:
_____
_____
_____
_____
_____

WEIGHT: _____ *LBS*
_____ *AM/PM*

DATE

TIME

BODY AREA

EXERCISE	SET 1	SET 2	SET 3	SET 4	SET 5	SET 6
	REPS/LBS	REPS/LBS	REPS/LBS	REPS/LBS	REPS/LBS	REPS/LBS

CARDIO EXERCISE:

NOTES:

DATE:

_____

BREAKFAST:

_____
At: _____

LUNCH:

_____
At: _____

DINNER:

_____
At: _____

SNACKS:
At: _____
_____
At: _____
_____
At: _____
_____
At: _____
_____

NOTES:

_____

_____

_____

_____

_____

WEIGHT: _____ *LBS*
                   _____ *AM/PM*

DATE **TIME** **BODY AREA**

EXERCISE	SET 1 REPS/LBS	SET 2 REPS/LBS	SET 3 REPS/LBS	SET 4 REPS/LBS	SET 5 REPS/LBS	SET 6 REPS/LBS

CARDIO EXERCISE:

_____

_____

_____

_____

NOTES:

_____

_____

_____

_____

DATE:

_____

BREAKFAST:

At: _____

LUNCH:

At: _____

DINNER:

At: _____

SNACKS:
At: _____

At: _____

At: _____

At: _____

NOTES:

_____

_____

_____

_____

_____

WEIGHT: _____ *LBS*
                 _____ *AM/PM*

DATE

TIME

BODY AREA

_____

_____

_____

EXERCISE	SET 1	SET 2	SET 3	SET 4	SET 5	SET 6
	REPS/LBS	REPS/LBS	REPS/LBS	REPS/LBS	REPS/LBS	REPS/LBS

CARDIO EXERCISE:

_____

_____

_____

_____

NOTES:

_____

_____

_____

_____

DATE:

_____

BREAKFAST:

_____

At: _____

LUNCH:

_____

At: _____

DINNER:

_____

At: _____

SNACKS:
At: _____

At: _____

At: _____

At: _____

NOTES:

_____

_____

_____

_____

_____

WEIGHT: _____ *LBS*
              _____ *AM/PM*

DATE   **TIME**   **BODY AREA**

_____   _____   _____

EXERCISE	SET 1	SET 2	SET 3	SET 4	SET 5	SET 6
	REPS/LBS	REPS/LBS	REPS/LBS	REPS/LBS	REPS/LBS	REPS/LBS

CARDIO EXERCISE:

_____

_____

_____

_____

NOTES:

_____

_____

_____

_____

DATE: _____

BREAKFAST:

_____

At: _____

_____

LUNCH:

_____

At: _____

_____

DINNER:

_____

At: _____

_____

SNACKS:

At: _____

_____

At: _____

_____

At: _____

_____

At: _____

_____

NOTES:

_____

_____

_____

_____

_____

WEIGHT: _____ *LBS*

_____ *AM/PM*

DATE _____

TIME _____

BODY AREA _____

EXERCISE	SET 1	SET 2	SET 3	SET 4	SET 5	SET 6
	REPS/LBS	REPS/LBS	REPS/LBS	REPS/LBS	REPS/LBS	REPS/LBS

CARDIO EXERCISE:

_____

_____

_____

_____

NOTES:

_____

_____

_____

_____

DATE:

_____

BREAKFAST:

At: _____

_____

LUNCH:

At: _____

_____

DINNER:

At: _____

_____

SNACKS:

At: _____

At: _____

At: _____

At: _____

NOTES:

_____

_____

_____

_____

_____

WEIGHT:　　_____ *LBS*

　　　　　　_____ *AM/PM*

DATE   **TIME**   **BODY AREA**

_____   _____   _____

EXERCISE	SET 1	SET 2	SET 3	SET 4	SET 5	SET 6
	REPS/LBS	REPS/LBS	REPS/LBS	REPS/LBS	REPS/LBS	REPS/LBS

CARDIO EXERCISE:

_____

_____

_____

_____

NOTES:

_____

_____

_____

_____

DATE:
_____

BREAKFAST:

At: _____
_____

_____

LUNCH:

At: _____
_____

_____

DINNER:

At: _____
_____

_____

SNACKS:
At: _____
_____

At: _____
_____

At: _____
_____

At: _____
_____

NOTES:

_____

_____

_____

_____

_____

WEIGHT: _____ *LBS*
              _____ *AM/PM*

DATE   TIME   BODY AREA

_____   _____   _____

EXERCISE	SET 1	SET 2	SET 3	SET 4	SET 5	SET 6
	REPS/LBS	REPS/LBS	REPS/LBS	REPS/LBS	REPS/LBS	REPS/LBS

CARDIO EXERCISE:

_____

_____

_____

_____

NOTES:

_____

_____

_____

_____

DATE:
_____

BREAKFAST:
_____
At: _____
_____

LUNCH:
_____
At: _____
_____

DINNER:
_____
At: _____
_____

SNACKS:
At: _____
_____
At: _____
_____
At: _____
_____
At: _____
_____

NOTES:

_____
_____
_____
_____
_____

WEIGHT: _____ LBS
_____ AM/PM

DATE

TIME

BODY AREA

EXERCISE	SET 1	SET 2	SET 3	SET 4	SET 5	SET 6
	REPS/LBS	REPS/LBS	REPS/LBS	REPS/LBS	REPS/LBS	REPS/LBS

CARDIO EXERCISE:

_____

_____

_____

_____

NOTES:

_____

_____

_____

_____

DATE:

BREAKFAST:

At: _____

LUNCH:

At: _____

DINNER:

At: _____

SNACKS:
At: _____

At: _____

At: _____

At: _____

NOTES:

WEIGHT: _____ *LBS*
                 _____ *AM/PM*

DATE **TIME** **BODY AREA**

_____ _____ _____

EXERCISE	SET 1	SET 2	SET 3	SET 4	SET 5	SET 6
	REPS/LBS	REPS/LBS	REPS/LBS	REPS/LBS	REPS/LBS	REPS/LBS

CARDIO EXERCISE:

_____

_____

_____

_____

NOTES:

_____

_____

_____

_____

DATE:
_____

BREAKFAST:

At: _____ _____

_____

LUNCH:

At: _____ _____

_____

DINNER:

At: _____ _____

_____

SNACKS:
At: _____ _____

At: _____ _____

At: _____ _____

At: _____ _____

NOTES:

_____

_____

_____

_____

_____

WEIGHT: _____ *LBS*
              _____ *AM/PM*

DATE

TIME

BODY AREA

EXERCISE	SET 1 REPS/LBS	SET 2 REPS/LBS	SET 3 REPS/LBS	SET 4 REPS/LBS	SET 5 REPS/LBS	SET 6 REPS/LBS

CARDIO EXERCISE:

_____

_____

_____

_____

NOTES:

_____

_____

_____

_____

DATE:
_____

BREAKFAST:

At: _____
_____

LUNCH:

At: _____
_____

DINNER:

At: _____
_____

SNACKS:
At: _____

At: _____

At: _____

At: _____

NOTES:

_____

_____

_____

_____

_____

WEIGHT: _____ *LBS*
                 _____ *AM/PM*

DATE   TIME   BODY AREA

_____   _____   _____

EXERCISE	SET 1	SET 2	SET 3	SET 4	SET 5	SET 6
	REPS/LBS	REPS/LBS	REPS/LBS	REPS/LBS	REPS/LBS	REPS/LBS

CARDIO EXERCISE:

_____

_____

_____

_____

NOTES:

_____

_____

_____

_____

DATE:
_____

BREAKFAST:

At: _____ _____

LUNCH:

At: _____ _____

DINNER:

At: _____ _____

SNACKS:
At: _____ _____

At: _____ _____

At: _____ _____

At: _____ _____

NOTES:

_____

_____

_____

_____

_____

WEIGHT: _____ *LBS*
              _____ *AM/PM*

DATE   TIME   BODY AREA

EXERCISE	SET 1	SET 2	SET 3	SET 4	SET 5	SET 6
	REPS/LBS	REPS/LBS	REPS/LBS	REPS/LBS	REPS/LBS	REPS/LBS

CARDIO EXERCISE:

_____

_____

_____

_____

NOTES:

_____

_____

_____

_____

DATE:
_____

BREAKFAST:

At: _____
_____

LUNCH:

At: _____
_____

DINNER:

At: _____
_____

SNACKS:
At: _____
_____

At: _____
_____

At: _____
_____

At: _____
_____

NOTES:

_____

_____

_____

_____

_____

WEIGHT: _____ *LBS*
                 _____ *AM/PM*

DATE   TIME   BODY AREA

_____   _____   _____

EXERCISE	SET 1 REPS/LBS	SET 2 REPS/LBS	SET 3 REPS/LBS	SET 4 REPS/LBS	SET 5 REPS/LBS	SET 6 REPS/LBS

CARDIO EXERCISE:

_____

_____

_____

_____

NOTES:

_____

_____

_____

_____

DATE:

_____

BREAKFAST:

_____
At: _____

_____

LUNCH:

_____
At: _____

_____

DINNER:

_____
At: _____

_____

SNACKS:
At: _____

_____
At: _____

_____
At: _____

_____
At: _____

_____

NOTES:

_____

_____

_____

_____

_____

WEIGHT: _____ **LBS**
                   _____ **AM/PM**

DATE   TIME   BODY AREA
_____   _____   _____

| EXERCISE | SET 1 | SET 2 | SET 3 | SET 4 | SET 5 | SET 6 |
	REPS/LBS	REPS/LBS	REPS/LBS	REPS/LBS	REPS/LBS	REPS/LBS

CARDIO EXERCISE:
_____
_____
_____
_____

NOTES:
_____
_____
_____
_____

DATE:

_____

BREAKFAST:

At: _____ _____

LUNCH:

At: _____ _____

DINNER:

At: _____ _____

SNACKS:
At: _____ _____

At: _____ _____

At: _____ _____

At: _____ _____

NOTES:

_____

_____

_____

_____

_____

WEIGHT: _____ *LBS*
                 _____ *AM/PM*

DATE   TIME   BODY AREA
_____   _____   _____

EXERCISE	SET 1	SET 2	SET 3	SET 4	SET 5	SET 6
	REPS/LBS	REPS/LBS	REPS/LBS	REPS/LBS	REPS/LBS	REPS/LBS

CARDIO EXERCISE:

_____
_____
_____
_____

NOTES:

_____
_____
_____
_____

DATE:
_____

BREAKFAST:

At: _____
_____

LUNCH:

At: _____
_____

DINNER:

At: _____
_____

SNACKS:
At: _____

At: _____

At: _____

At: _____

NOTES:

_____

_____

_____

_____

_____

WEIGHT: _____ *LBS*
                          _____ *AM/PM*

DATE   **TIME**   **BODY AREA**

_____   _____   _____

EXERCISE	SET 1	SET 2	SET 3	SET 4	SET 5	SET 6
	REPS/LBS	REPS/LBS	REPS/LBS	REPS/LBS	REPS/LBS	REPS/LBS

CARDIO EXERCISE:

_____

_____

_____

_____

NOTES:

_____

_____

_____

_____

DATE:

_____

BREAKFAST:

At: _____

LUNCH:

At: _____

DINNER:

At: _____

SNACKS:
At: _____

At: _____

At: _____

At: _____

NOTES:

_____

_____

_____

_____

_____

WEIGHT: _____ *LBS*
                 _____ *AM/PM*

DATE   TIME   BODY AREA

_____   _____   _____

EXERCISE	SET 1	SET 2	SET 3	SET 4	SET 5	SET 6
	REPS/LBS	REPS/LBS	REPS/LBS	REPS/LBS	REPS/LBS	REPS/LBS

CARDIO EXERCISE:

_____

_____

_____

_____

NOTES:

_____

_____

_____

_____

DATE:

BREAKFAST:

At: _____

LUNCH:

At: _____

DINNER:

At: _____

SNACKS:
At: _____

At: _____

At: _____

At: _____

NOTES:

WEIGHT: _____ *LBS*
_____ *AM/PM*

DATE

TIME

BODY AREA

EXERCISE	SET 1 REPS/LBS	SET 2 REPS/LBS	SET 3 REPS/LBS	SET 4 REPS/LBS	SET 5 REPS/LBS	SET 6 REPS/LBS

CARDIO EXERCISE:

_____

_____

_____

_____

NOTES:

_____

_____

_____

_____

DATE:

_____

BREAKFAST:

_____

At: _____

LUNCH:

_____

At: _____

DINNER:

_____

At: _____

SNACKS:
At: _____

_____

At: _____

_____

At: _____

_____

At: _____

NOTES:

_____

_____

_____

_____

_____

WEIGHT: _____ *LBS*
                 _____ *AM/PM*

DATE _____

TIME _____

BODY AREA _____

EXERCISE	SET 1 REPS/LBS	SET 2 REPS/LBS	SET 3 REPS/LBS	SET 4 REPS/LBS	SET 5 REPS/LBS	SET 6 REPS/LBS

CARDIO EXERCISE:

_____

_____

_____

_____

NOTES:

_____

_____

_____

_____

DATE:

_____

BREAKFAST:

At: _____

LUNCH:

At: _____

DINNER:

At: _____

SNACKS:

At: _____

At: _____

At: _____

At: _____

NOTES:

_____

_____

_____

_____

_____

WEIGHT: _____ *LBS*

     _____ *AM/PM*

DATE   TIME   BODY AREA

_____   _____   _____

EXERCISE	SET 1 REPS/LBS	SET 2 REPS/LBS	SET 3 REPS/LBS	SET 4 REPS/LBS	SET 5 REPS/LBS	SET 6 REPS/LBS

CARDIO EXERCISE:

_____

_____

_____

_____

NOTES:

_____

_____

_____

_____

DATE:

BREAKFAST:

At: _____

LUNCH:

At: _____

DINNER:

At: _____

SNACKS:
At: _____

At: _____

At: _____

At: _____

NOTES:

WEIGHT: _____ *LBS*
_____ *AM/PM*

DATE

TIME

BODY AREA

EXERCISE	SET 1	SET 2	SET 3	SET 4	SET 5	SET 6
	REPS/LBS	REPS/LBS	REPS/LBS	REPS/LBS	REPS/LBS	REPS/LBS

CARDIO EXERCISE:

_____

_____

_____

_____

NOTES:

_____

_____

_____

_____

DATE:
_____

BREAKFAST:
_____
At: _____
_____

LUNCH:
_____
At: _____
_____

DINNER:
_____
At: _____
_____

SNACKS:
At: _____
_____
At: _____
_____
At: _____
_____
At: _____
_____

NOTES:

_____

_____

_____

_____

_____

WEIGHT: _____ *LBS*
                 _____ *AM/PM*

DATE   TIME   BODY AREA

EXERCISE	SET 1 REPS/LBS	SET 2 REPS/LBS	SET 3 REPS/LBS	SET 4 REPS/LBS	SET 5 REPS/LBS	SET 6 REPS/LBS

CARDIO EXERCISE:

_____

_____

_____

_____

NOTES:

_____

_____

_____

_____

DATE:

BREAKFAST:

At: _____

LUNCH:

At: _____

DINNER:

At: _____

SNACKS:
At: _____

At: _____

At: _____

At: _____

NOTES:

WEIGHT: _____ *LBS*
                _____ *AM/PM*

DATE

_____

TIME

_____

BODY AREA

_____

EXERCISE	SET 1	SET 2	SET 3	SET 4	SET 5	SET 6
	REPS/LBS	REPS/LBS	REPS/LBS	REPS/LBS	REPS/LBS	REPS/LBS

CARDIO EXERCISE:

_____

_____

_____

_____

NOTES:

_____

_____

_____

_____

DATE:

_____

BREAKFAST:

_____

At: _____ _____

LUNCH:

_____

At: _____ _____

DINNER:

_____

At: _____ _____

SNACKS:
At: _____ _____

At: _____ _____

At: _____ _____

At: _____ _____

NOTES:

_____

_____

_____

_____

_____

WEIGHT: _____ *LBS*

_____ *AM/PM*

DATE

TIME

BODY AREA

_____

_____

_____

EXERCISE	SET 1	SET 2	SET 3	SET 4	SET 5	SET 6
	REPS/LBS	REPS/LBS	REPS/LBS	REPS/LBS	REPS/LBS	REPS/LBS

CARDIO EXERCISE:

_____

_____

_____

_____

NOTES:

_____

_____

_____

_____

DATE:
_____

BREAKFAST:
_____
At: _____
_____

LUNCH:
_____
At: _____
_____

DINNER:
_____
At: _____
_____

SNACKS:
At: _____
_____
At: _____
_____
At: _____
_____
At: _____

NOTES:

_____
_____
_____
_____
_____

WEIGHT: _____ *LBS*
                 _____ *AM/PM*

DATE   TIME   BODY AREA

_____   _____   _____

EXERCISE	SET 1	SET 2	SET 3	SET 4	SET 5	SET 6
	REPS/LBS	REPS/LBS	REPS/LBS	REPS/LBS	REPS/LBS	REPS/LBS

CARDIO EXERCISE:

_____

_____

_____

_____

NOTES:

_____

_____

_____

_____

DATE:

_____

BREAKFAST:

At: _____

LUNCH:

At: _____

DINNER:

At: _____

SNACKS:

At: _____

At: _____

At: _____

At: _____

NOTES:

_____

_____

_____

_____

_____

WEIGHT: _____ *LBS*

                _____ *AM/PM*

DATE _____   TIME _____   BODY AREA _____

EXERCISE	SET 1 REPS/LBS	SET 2 REPS/LBS	SET 3 REPS/LBS	SET 4 REPS/LBS	SET 5 REPS/LBS	SET 6 REPS/LBS

CARDIO EXERCISE:

_____
_____
_____
_____

NOTES:

_____
_____
_____
_____

DATE: _____

BREAKFAST:
_____
At: _____
_____

LUNCH:
_____
At: _____
_____

DINNER:
_____
At: _____
_____

SNACKS:
At: _____
_____
At: _____
_____
At: _____
_____
At: _____
_____

NOTES:
_____
_____
_____
_____
_____

WEIGHT: _____ *LBS*
             _____ *AM/PM*

DATE   TIME   BODY AREA

EXERCISE	SET 1 REPS/LBS	SET 2 REPS/LBS	SET 3 REPS/LBS	SET 4 REPS/LBS	SET 5 REPS/LBS	SET 6 REPS/LBS

CARDIO EXERCISE:

_____

_____

_____

_____

NOTES:

_____

_____

_____

_____

DATE:

_____

BREAKFAST:

At: _____

LUNCH:

At: _____

DINNER:

At: _____

SNACKS:
At: _____

At: _____

At: _____

At: _____

NOTES:

_____

_____

_____

_____

_____

WEIGHT: _____ *LBS*
             _____ *AM/PM*

DATE _____ TIME _____ BODY AREA _____

EXERCISE	SET 1 REPS/LBS	SET 2 REPS/LBS	SET 3 REPS/LBS	SET 4 REPS/LBS	SET 5 REPS/LBS	SET 6 REPS/LBS

CARDIO EXERCISE:

_____

_____

_____

_____

NOTES:

_____

_____

_____

_____

DATE:
_____

BREAKFAST:
_____
At: _____

LUNCH:
_____
At: _____

DINNER:
_____
At: _____

SNACKS:
At: _____
_____
At: _____
_____
At: _____
_____
At: _____
_____

NOTES:

_____

_____

_____

_____

_____

WEIGHT: _____ *LBS*
_____ *AM/PM*

DATE _____ TIME _____ BODY AREA _____

EXERCISE	SET 1	SET 2	SET 3	SET 4	SET 5	SET 6
	REPS/LBS	REPS/LBS	REPS/LBS	REPS/LBS	REPS/LBS	REPS/LBS

CARDIO EXERCISE:

_____

_____

_____

_____

NOTES:

_____

_____

_____

_____

DATE:

_____

BREAKFAST:

At: _____

_____

LUNCH:

At: _____

_____

DINNER:

At: _____

_____

SNACKS:
At: _____

At: _____

At: _____

At: _____

NOTES:

_____

_____

_____

_____

_____

WEIGHT: _____ *LBS*
                 _____ *AM/PM*

DATE   TIME   BODY AREA

_____   _____   _____

EXERCISE	SET 1 REPS/LBS	SET 2 REPS/LBS	SET 3 REPS/LBS	SET 4 REPS/LBS	SET 5 REPS/LBS	SET 6 REPS/LBS

CARDIO EXERCISE:

_____

_____

_____

_____

NOTES:

_____

_____

_____

_____

DATE:

_____

BREAKFAST:

At: _____   _____

_____

LUNCH:

At: _____   _____

_____

DINNER:

At: _____   _____

_____

SNACKS:
At: _____   _____

At: _____   _____

At: _____   _____

At: _____   _____

NOTES:

_____

_____

_____

_____

_____

WEIGHT: _____ *LBS*
                 _____ *AM/PM*

DATE   TIME   BODY AREA

_____   _____   _____

EXERCISE	SET 1	SET 2	SET 3	SET 4	SET 5	SET 6
	REPS/LBS	REPS/LBS	REPS/LBS	REPS/LBS	REPS/LBS	REPS/LBS

CARDIO EXERCISE:

_____

_____

_____

_____

NOTES:

_____

_____

_____

_____

DATE: _____

BREAKFAST:

_____
At: _____
_____

LUNCH:

_____
At: _____
_____

DINNER:

_____
At: _____
_____

SNACKS:
At: _____
_____
At: _____
_____
At: _____
_____
At: _____
_____

NOTES:

_____
_____
_____
_____
_____

WEIGHT: _____ **LBS**
_____ **AM/PM**

DATE _____

TIME _____

BODY AREA _____

EXERCISE	SET 1	SET 2	SET 3	SET 4	SET 5	SET 6
	REPS/LBS	REPS/LBS	REPS/LBS	REPS/LBS	REPS/LBS	REPS/LBS

CARDIO EXERCISE:

_____

_____

_____

_____

NOTES:

_____

_____

_____

_____

DATE:
_____

BREAKFAST:

At: _____ _____
_____

LUNCH:

At: _____ _____
_____

DINNER:

At: _____ _____
_____

SNACKS:
At: _____ _____

At: _____ _____

At: _____ _____

At: _____ _____

NOTES:

_____
_____
_____
_____
_____

WEIGHT: _____ *LBS*
               _____ *AM/PM*

DATE   TIME   BODY AREA

_____   _____   _____

EXERCISE	SET 1	SET 2	SET 3	SET 4	SET 5	SET 6
	REPS/LBS	REPS/LBS	REPS/LBS	REPS/LBS	REPS/LBS	REPS/LBS

CARDIO EXERCISE:

_____

_____

_____

_____

NOTES:

_____

_____

_____

_____

DATE:

_____

BREAKFAST:

_____
At: _____

LUNCH:

_____
At: _____

DINNER:

_____
At: _____

SNACKS:
At: _____

_____
At: _____

_____
At: _____

_____
At: _____

NOTES:

_____

_____

_____

_____

_____

WEIGHT: _____ *LBS*
                 _____ *AM/PM*

DATE   TIME   BODY AREA

_____   _____   _____

EXERCISE	SET 1	SET 2	SET 3	SET 4	SET 5	SET 6
	REPS/LBS	REPS/LBS	REPS/LBS	REPS/LBS	REPS/LBS	REPS/LBS

CARDIO EXERCISE:

_____

_____

_____

_____

NOTES:

_____

_____

_____

_____

DATE: _____

BREAKFAST:

At: _____

LUNCH:

At: _____

DINNER:

At: _____

SNACKS:
At: _____

At: _____

At: _____

At: _____

NOTES:

_____

_____

_____

_____

_____

WEIGHT: _____ *LBS*
          _____ *AM/PM*

DATE _____ TIME _____ BODY AREA _____

EXERCISE	SET 1	SET 2	SET 3	SET 4	SET 5	SET 6
	REPS/LBS	REPS/LBS	REPS/LBS	REPS/LBS	REPS/LBS	REPS/LBS

CARDIO EXERCISE:

_____
_____
_____
_____

NOTES:

_____
_____
_____
_____

DATE:

_____

BREAKFAST:

At: _____ _____

_____

LUNCH:

At: _____ _____

_____

DINNER:

At: _____ _____

_____

SNACKS:
At: _____ _____

At: _____ _____

At: _____ _____

At: _____ _____

NOTES:

_____

_____

_____

_____

_____

WEIGHT:　　　_____ *LBS*
　　　　　　　_____ *AM/PM*

DATE   TIME   BODY AREA

_____   _____   _____

EXERCISE	SET 1	SET 2	SET 3	SET 4	SET 5	SET 6
	REPS/LBS	REPS/LBS	REPS/LBS	REPS/LBS	REPS/LBS	REPS/LBS

CARDIO EXERCISE:

_____

_____

_____

_____

NOTES:

_____

_____

_____

_____

DATE:
_____

BREAKFAST:
_____
At: _____
_____

LUNCH:
_____
At: _____
_____

DINNER:
_____
At: _____
_____

SNACKS:
At: _____
_____
At: _____
_____
At: _____
_____

NOTES:

_____

_____

_____

_____

_____

WEIGHT: _____ *LBS*
              _____ *AM/PM*

DATE   TIME   BODY AREA

_____   _____   _____

EXERCISE	SET 1	SET 2	SET 3	SET 4	SET 5	SET 6
	REPS/LBS	REPS/LBS	REPS/LBS	REPS/LBS	REPS/LBS	REPS/LBS

CARDIO EXERCISE:

_____

_____

_____

_____

NOTES:

_____

_____

_____

_____

DATE:
_____

BREAKFAST:
_____
At: _____
_____

LUNCH:
_____
At: _____
_____

DINNER:
_____
At: _____
_____

SNACKS:
At: _____
_____
At: _____
_____
At: _____
_____
At: _____
_____

NOTES:

_____
_____
_____
_____
_____

WEIGHT: _____ *LBS*
              _____ *AM/PM*

DATE   TIME   BODY AREA

_____   _____   _____

EXERCISE	SET 1	SET 2	SET 3	SET 4	SET 5	SET 6
	REPS/LBS	REPS/LBS	REPS/LBS	REPS/LBS	REPS/LBS	REPS/LBS

CARDIO EXERCISE:

_____

_____

_____

_____

NOTES:

_____

_____

_____

_____

DATE:

BREAKFAST:

At: _____

LUNCH:

At: _____

DINNER:

At: _____

SNACKS:
At: _____

At: _____

At: _____

At: _____

NOTES:

WEIGHT:　　_____ *LBS*
　　　　　　　_____ *AM/PM*

DATE   TIME   BODY AREA

EXERCISE	SET 1	SET 2	SET 3	SET 4	SET 5	SET 6
	REPS/LBS	REPS/LBS	REPS/LBS	REPS/LBS	REPS/LBS	REPS/LBS

CARDIO EXERCISE:

_____

_____

_____

_____

NOTES:

_____

_____

_____

_____

DATE:
_____

BREAKFAST:

At: _____
_____

LUNCH:

At: _____
_____

DINNER:

At: _____
_____

SNACKS:
At: _____

At: _____

At: _____

At: _____

NOTES:

_____

_____

_____

_____

_____

WEIGHT: _____ *LBS*
                 _____ *AM/PM*

DATE   TIME   BODY AREA

_____   _____   _____

EXERCISE	SET 1	SET 2	SET 3	SET 4	SET 5	SET 6
	REPS/LBS	REPS/LBS	REPS/LBS	REPS/LBS	REPS/LBS	REPS/LBS

CARDIO EXERCISE:

_____
_____
_____
_____

NOTES:

_____
_____
_____
_____

DATE:

_____

BREAKFAST:

At: _____

_____

LUNCH:

At: _____

_____

DINNER:

At: _____

_____

SNACKS:
At: _____

At: _____

At: _____

At: _____

NOTES:

_____

_____

_____

_____

_____

WEIGHT: _____ **LBS**
               _____ **AM/PM**

DATE _____   TIME _____   BODY AREA _____

EXERCISE	SET 1	SET 2	SET 3	SET 4	SET 5	SET 6
	REPS/LBS	REPS/LBS	REPS/LBS	REPS/LBS	REPS/LBS	REPS/LBS

CARDIO EXERCISE:

_____

_____

_____

_____

NOTES:

_____

_____

_____

_____

DATE: _____

BREAKFAST:

At: _____ _____

LUNCH:

At: _____ _____

DINNER:

At: _____ _____

SNACKS:
At: _____ _____

At: _____ _____

At: _____ _____

At: _____ _____

NOTES:

_____

_____

_____

_____

_____

WEIGHT: _____ *LBS*
_____ *AM/PM*

DATE

TIME

BODY AREA

EXERCISE	SET 1 REPS/LBS	SET 2 REPS/LBS	SET 3 REPS/LBS	SET 4 REPS/LBS	SET 5 REPS/LBS	SET 6 REPS/LBS

CARDIO EXERCISE:

_____

_____

_____

_____

NOTES:

_____

_____

_____

_____

DATE:

_____

BREAKFAST:

At: _____

_____

LUNCH:

At: _____

_____

DINNER:

At: _____

_____

SNACKS:

At: _____

_____

At: _____

_____

At: _____

_____

At: _____

_____

NOTES:

_____

_____

_____

_____

_____

WEIGHT: _____ *LBS*
              _____ *AM/PM*

DATE _____

TIME _____

BODY AREA _____

EXERCISE	SET 1 REPS/LBS	SET 2 REPS/LBS	SET 3 REPS/LBS	SET 4 REPS/LBS	SET 5 REPS/LBS	SET 6 REPS/LBS

CARDIO EXERCISE:

_____

_____

_____

_____

NOTES:

_____

_____

_____

_____

DATE:

_____

BREAKFAST:

At: _____

LUNCH:

At: _____

DINNER:

At: _____

SNACKS:
At: _____

At: _____

At: _____

At: _____

NOTES:

_____

_____

_____

_____

_____

WEIGHT: _____ LBS
_____ AM/PM

DATE _____ TIME _____ BODY AREA _____

EXERCISE	SET 1 REPS/LBS	SET 2 REPS/LBS	SET 3 REPS/LBS	SET 4 REPS/LBS	SET 5 REPS/LBS	SET 6 REPS/LBS

CARDIO EXERCISE:

_____

_____

_____

_____

NOTES:

_____

_____

_____

_____

DATE:
_____

BREAKFAST:
_____
At: _____
_____

LUNCH:
_____
At: _____
_____

DINNER:
_____
At: _____
_____

SNACKS:
At: _____
_____
At: _____
_____
At: _____
_____
At: _____

NOTES:

_____
_____
_____
_____
_____

WEIGHT: _____ *LBS*
                 _____ *AM/PM*

DATE   **TIME**   **BODY AREA**

    _____   _____   _____

EXERCISE	SET 1	SET 2	SET 3	SET 4	SET 5	SET 6
	REPS/LBS	REPS/LBS	REPS/LBS	REPS/LBS	REPS/LBS	REPS/LBS

CARDIO EXERCISE:

_____

_____

_____

_____

NOTES:

_____

_____

_____

_____

DATE:

_____

BREAKFAST:

_____
At: _____

LUNCH:

_____
At: _____

DINNER:

_____
At: _____

SNACKS:
At: _____

_____
At: _____

_____
At: _____

_____
At: _____

NOTES:

_____

_____

_____

_____

_____

WEIGHT: _____ **LBS**
                  _____ **AM/PM**

DATE   TIME   BODY AREA

_____   _____   _____

EXERCISE	SET 1	SET 2	SET 3	SET 4	SET 5	SET 6
	REPS/LBS	REPS/LBS	REPS/LBS	REPS/LBS	REPS/LBS	REPS/LBS

CARDIO EXERCISE:

_____

_____

_____

_____

NOTES:

_____

_____

_____

_____

DATE:

_____

BREAKFAST:

_____

At: _____

_____

LUNCH:

_____

At: _____

_____

DINNER:

_____

At: _____

_____

SNACKS:

At: _____

_____

At: _____

_____

At: _____

_____

At: _____

_____

NOTES:

_____

_____

_____

_____

_____

WEIGHT: _____ **LBS**
_____ **AM/PM**

DATE   TIME   BODY AREA

_____   _____   _____

EXERCISE	SET 1	SET 2	SET 3	SET 4	SET 5	SET 6
	REPS/LBS	REPS/LBS	REPS/LBS	REPS/LBS	REPS/LBS	REPS/LBS

CARDIO EXERCISE:

_____

_____

_____

_____

NOTES:

_____

_____

_____

_____

DATE:

BREAKFAST:

At: _____

LUNCH:

At: _____

DINNER:

At: _____

SNACKS:
At: _____

At: _____

At: _____

At: _____

NOTES:

WEIGHT: _____ *LBS*
                 _____ *AM/PM*

DATE

TIME

BODY AREA

EXERCISE	SET 1 REPS/LBS	SET 2 REPS/LBS	SET 3 REPS/LBS	SET 4 REPS/LBS	SET 5 REPS/LBS	SET 6 REPS/LBS

CARDIO EXERCISE:

_____

_____

_____

_____

NOTES:

_____

_____

_____

_____

DATE:

BREAKFAST:

At: _____

LUNCH:

At: _____

DINNER:

At: _____

SNACKS:
At: _____

At: _____

At: _____

At: _____

NOTES:

WEIGHT: _____ *LBS*
_____ *AM/PM*

DATE

TIME

BODY AREA

EXERCISE	SET 1 REPS/LBS	SET 2 REPS/LBS	SET 3 REPS/LBS	SET 4 REPS/LBS	SET 5 REPS/LBS	SET 6 REPS/LBS

CARDIO EXERCISE:

NOTES:

DATE:
_____

BREAKFAST:
_____
At: _____
_____

LUNCH:
_____
At: _____
_____

DINNER:
_____
At: _____
_____

SNACKS:
At: _____
_____
At: _____
_____
At: _____
_____
At: _____
_____

NOTES:

_____
_____
_____
_____
_____

WEIGHT: _____ *LBS*
               _____ *AM/PM*

DATE

TIME

BODY AREA

_____

_____

_____

EXERCISE	SET 1 REPS/LBS	SET 2 REPS/LBS	SET 3 REPS/LBS	SET 4 REPS/LBS	SET 5 REPS/LBS	SET 6 REPS/LBS

CARDIO EXERCISE:

_____

_____

_____

_____

NOTES:

_____

_____

_____

_____

DATE:
_____

BREAKFAST:

At: _____ _____

LUNCH:

At: _____ _____

DINNER:

At: _____ _____

SNACKS:
At: _____ _____

At: _____ _____

At: _____ _____

At: _____ _____

NOTES:

_____

_____

_____

_____

_____

WEIGHT: _____ *LBS*
                 _____ *AM/PM*

DATE

TIME

BODY AREA

EXERCISE	SET 1	SET 2	SET 3	SET 4	SET 5	SET 6
	REPS/LBS	REPS/LBS	REPS/LBS	REPS/LBS	REPS/LBS	REPS/LBS

CARDIO EXERCISE:

NOTES:

DATE:
_____

BREAKFAST:

At: _____
_____

LUNCH:

At: _____
_____

DINNER:

At: _____
_____

SNACKS:
At: _____
_____

At: _____
_____

At: _____
_____

NOTES:

_____

_____

_____

_____

_____

WEIGHT: _____ *LBS*
                 _____ *AM/PM*

DATE   TIME   BODY AREA

_____   _____   _____

EXERCISE	SET 1	SET 2	SET 3	SET 4	SET 5	SET 6
	REPS/LBS	REPS/LBS	REPS/LBS	REPS/LBS	REPS/LBS	REPS/LBS

CARDIO EXERCISE:

_____

_____

_____

_____

NOTES:

_____

_____

_____

_____

DATE:

_____

BREAKFAST:

_____

At: _____

_____

LUNCH:

_____

At: _____

_____

DINNER:

_____

At: _____

_____

SNACKS:

At: _____

_____

At: _____

_____

At: _____

_____

At: _____

_____

NOTES:

_____

_____

_____

_____

_____

WEIGHT: _____ *LBS*

                 _____ *AM/PM*

DATE _____ TIME _____ BODY AREA _____

EXERCISE	SET 1 REPS/LBS	SET 2 REPS/LBS	SET 3 REPS/LBS	SET 4 REPS/LBS	SET 5 REPS/LBS	SET 6 REPS/LBS

CARDIO EXERCISE:

_____

_____

_____

_____

NOTES:

_____

_____

_____

_____

DATE:
_____

BREAKFAST:
_____
At: _____
_____

LUNCH:
_____
At: _____
_____

DINNER:
_____
At: _____
_____

SNACKS:
At: _____
_____
At: _____
_____
At: _____
_____
At: _____
_____

NOTES:
_____
_____
_____
_____
_____

WEIGHT: _____ *LBS*
                 _____ *AM/PM*

DATE _____ TIME _____ BODY AREA _____

EXERCISE	SET 1 REPS/LBS	SET 2 REPS/LBS	SET 3 REPS/LBS	SET 4 REPS/LBS	SET 5 REPS/LBS	SET 6 REPS/LBS

CARDIO EXERCISE:

_____

_____

_____

_____

NOTES:

_____

_____

_____

_____

DATE:

_____

BREAKFAST:

At: _____ _____

_____

LUNCH:

At: _____ _____

_____

DINNER:

At: _____ _____

_____

SNACKS:
At: _____ _____

At: _____ _____

At: _____ _____

At: _____ _____

NOTES:

_____

_____

_____

_____

_____

WEIGHT: _____ *LBS*
                 _____ *AM/PM*

DATE   TIME   BODY AREA

_____   _____   _____

EXERCISE	SET 1	SET 2	SET 3	SET 4	SET 5	SET 6
	REPS/LBS	REPS/LBS	REPS/LBS	REPS/LBS	REPS/LBS	REPS/LBS

CARDIO EXERCISE:

_____
_____
_____
_____

NOTES:

_____
_____
_____
_____

DATE:

_____

BREAKFAST:

_____

At: _____

LUNCH:

_____

At: _____

DINNER:

_____

At: _____

SNACKS:

At: _____

At: _____

At: _____

At: _____

NOTES:

_____

_____

_____

_____

_____

WEIGHT: _____ *LBS*
             _____ *AM/PM*

DATE   TIME   BODY AREA

_____   _____   _____

EXERCISE	SET 1	SET 2	SET 3	SET 4	SET 5	SET 6
	REPS/LBS	REPS/LBS	REPS/LBS	REPS/LBS	REPS/LBS	REPS/LBS

CARDIO EXERCISE:

_____
_____
_____
_____

NOTES:

_____
_____
_____
_____

DATE:
_____

BREAKFAST:
_____
At: _____
_____

LUNCH:
_____
At: _____
_____

DINNER:
_____
At: _____
_____

SNACKS:
At: _____
_____
At: _____
_____
At: _____
_____
At: _____
_____

NOTES:

_____
_____
_____
_____
_____

WEIGHT: _____ *LBS*
             _____ *AM/PM*

DATE   TIME   BODY AREA

_____   _____   _____

EXERCISE	SET 1	SET 2	SET 3	SET 4	SET 5	SET 6
	REPS/LBS	REPS/LBS	REPS/LBS	REPS/LBS	REPS/LBS	REPS/LBS

CARDIO EXERCISE:

_____

_____

_____

_____

NOTES:

_____

_____

_____

_____

DATE:
_____

BREAKFAST:
_____
At: _____
_____

LUNCH:
_____
At: _____
_____

DINNER:
_____
At: _____
_____

SNACKS:
At: _____
_____
At: _____
_____
At: _____
_____
At: _____
_____

NOTES:

_____
_____
_____
_____
_____

WEIGHT: _____ *LBS*
_____ *AM/PM*

DATE   TIME   BODY AREA

_____   _____   _____

EXERCISE	SET 1	SET 2	SET 3	SET 4	SET 5	SET 6
	REPS/LBS	REPS/LBS	REPS/LBS	REPS/LBS	REPS/LBS	REPS/LBS

CARDIO EXERCISE:

_____

_____

_____

_____

NOTES:

_____

_____

_____

_____

DATE: _____

BREAKFAST:

At: _____ _____

LUNCH:

At: _____ _____

DINNER:

At: _____ _____

SNACKS:
At: _____ _____

At: _____ _____

At: _____ _____

At: _____ _____

NOTES:

_____

_____

_____

_____

_____

WEIGHT: _____ *LBS*
_____ *AM/PM*

DATE   TIME   BODY AREA

_____   _____   _____

EXERCISE	SET 1	SET 2	SET 3	SET 4	SET 5	SET 6
	REPS/LBS	REPS/LBS	REPS/LBS	REPS/LBS	REPS/LBS	REPS/LBS

CARDIO EXERCISE:

_____
_____
_____
_____

NOTES:

_____
_____
_____
_____

DATE:

_____

BREAKFAST:

_____

At: _____

LUNCH:

_____

At: _____

DINNER:

_____

At: _____

SNACKS:
At: _____

_____

At: _____

_____

At: _____

_____

At: _____

NOTES:

_____

_____

_____

_____

_____

WEIGHT: _____ *LBS*
              _____ *AM/PM*

DATE   TIME   BODY AREA

_____   _____   _____

EXERCISE	SET 1	SET 2	SET 3	SET 4	SET 5	SET 6
	REPS/LBS	REPS/LBS	REPS/LBS	REPS/LBS	REPS/LBS	REPS/LBS

CARDIO EXERCISE:

_____
_____
_____
_____

NOTES:

_____
_____
_____
_____

DATE:

BREAKFAST:

At: _____

LUNCH:

At: _____

DINNER:

At: _____

SNACKS:

At: _____

At: _____

At: _____

At: _____

NOTES:

WEIGHT: _____ *LBS*
_____ *AM/PM*

DATE   TIME   BODY AREA

_____   _____   _____

EXERCISE	SET 1 REPS/LBS	SET 2 REPS/LBS	SET 3 REPS/LBS	SET 4 REPS/LBS	SET 5 REPS/LBS	SET 6 REPS/LBS

CARDIO EXERCISE:

_____

_____

_____

_____

NOTES:

_____

_____

_____

_____

DATE:

_____

BREAKFAST:

At: _____

LUNCH:

At: _____

DINNER:

At: _____

SNACKS:
At: _____

At: _____

At: _____

At: _____

NOTES:

_____

_____

_____

_____

_____

WEIGHT: _____ *LBS*
                 _____ *AM/PM*

DATE   TIME   BODY AREA

_____   _____   _____

EXERCISE	SET 1	SET 2	SET 3	SET 4	SET 5	SET 6
	REPS/LBS	REPS/LBS	REPS/LBS	REPS/LBS	REPS/LBS	REPS/LBS

CARDIO EXERCISE:

_____

_____

_____

_____

NOTES:

_____

_____

_____

_____

DATE:

_____

BREAKFAST:

_____
At: _____

_____

LUNCH:

_____
At: _____

_____

DINNER:

_____
At: _____

_____

SNACKS:
At: _____

_____
At: _____

_____
At: _____

_____
At: _____

_____

NOTES:

_____

_____

_____

_____

_____

WEIGHT: _____ *LBS*
                 _____ *AM/PM*

DATE   TIME   BODY AREA

EXERCISE	SET 1	SET 2	SET 3	SET 4	SET 5	SET 6
	REPS/LBS	REPS/LBS	REPS/LBS	REPS/LBS	REPS/LBS	REPS/LBS

CARDIO EXERCISE:

_____

_____

_____

_____

NOTES:

_____

_____

_____

_____

DATE:

_____

BREAKFAST:

At: _____

LUNCH:

At: _____

DINNER:

At: _____

SNACKS:
At: _____

At: _____

At: _____

At: _____

NOTES:

_____

_____

_____

_____

_____

WEIGHT: _____ *LBS*
              _____ *AM/PM*

DATE   TIME   BODY AREA

_____   _____   _____

EXERCISE	SET 1	SET 2	SET 3	SET 4	SET 5	SET 6
	REPS/LBS	REPS/LBS	REPS/LBS	REPS/LBS	REPS/LBS	REPS/LBS

CARDIO EXERCISE:

_____

_____

_____

_____

NOTES:

_____

_____

_____

_____

DATE:

_____

BREAKFAST:

_____

At: _____

LUNCH:

_____

At: _____

DINNER:

_____

At: _____

SNACKS:

At: _____

At: _____

At: _____

At: _____

NOTES:

_____

_____

_____

_____

_____

WEIGHT: _____ **LBS**

_____ **AM/PM**

DATE _____   **TIME** _____   **BODY AREA** _____

EXERCISE	SET 1 REPS/LBS	SET 2 REPS/LBS	SET 3 REPS/LBS	SET 4 REPS/LBS	SET 5 REPS/LBS	SET 6 REPS/LBS

CARDIO EXERCISE:

_____

_____

_____

NOTES:

_____

_____

_____

_____

DATE:

_____

BREAKFAST:
_____
At: _____
_____

LUNCH:
_____
At: _____
_____

DINNER:
_____
At: _____
_____

SNACKS:
At: _____
_____
At: _____
_____
At: _____
_____
At: _____

NOTES:

_____

_____

_____

_____

_____

WEIGHT:　　　_____ *LBS*
　　　　　　　_____ *AM/PM*

DATE   TIME   BODY AREA

_____   _____   _____

EXERCISE	SET 1	SET 2	SET 3	SET 4	SET 5	SET 6
	REPS/LBS	REPS/LBS	REPS/LBS	REPS/LBS	REPS/LBS	REPS/LBS

CARDIO EXERCISE:

_____

_____

_____

_____

NOTES:

_____

_____

_____

_____

DATE:

_____

BREAKFAST:

At: _____

LUNCH:

At: _____

DINNER:

At: _____

SNACKS:
At: _____

At: _____

At: _____

At: _____

NOTES:

_____

_____

_____

_____

_____

WEIGHT: _____ *LBS*
                 _____ *AM/PM*

DATE   TIME   BODY AREA
_____   _____   _____

EXERCISE	SET 1	SET 2	SET 3	SET 4	SET 5	SET 6
	REPS/LBS	REPS/LBS	REPS/LBS	REPS/LBS	REPS/LBS	REPS/LBS

CARDIO EXERCISE:
_____
_____
_____
_____

NOTES:
_____
_____
_____
_____

DATE:

_____

BREAKFAST:

_____
At: _____
_____

LUNCH:

_____
At: _____
_____

DINNER:

_____
At: _____
_____

SNACKS:
At: _____
_____
At: _____
_____
At: _____
_____
At: _____
_____

NOTES:

_____
_____
_____
_____
_____

WEIGHT: _____ *LBS*
                _____ *AM/PM*

DATE _____

TIME _____

BODY AREA _____

EXERCISE	SET 1 REPS/LBS	SET 2 REPS/LBS	SET 3 REPS/LBS	SET 4 REPS/LBS	SET 5 REPS/LBS	SET 6 REPS/LBS

CARDIO EXERCISE:

_____

_____

_____

_____

NOTES:

_____

_____

_____

_____

DATE:

_____

BREAKFAST:

At: _____

_____

_____

LUNCH:

At: _____

_____

_____

DINNER:

At: _____

_____

_____

SNACKS:

At: _____

_____

At: _____

_____

At: _____

_____

At: _____

_____

NOTES:

_____

_____

_____

_____

_____

WEIGHT: _____ *LBS*

_____ *AM/PM*

DATE _____   TIME _____   BODY AREA _____

EXERCISE	SET 1 REPS/LBS	SET 2 REPS/LBS	SET 3 REPS/LBS	SET 4 REPS/LBS	SET 5 REPS/LBS	SET 6 REPS/LBS

CARDIO EXERCISE:

_____
_____
_____
_____

NOTES:

_____
_____
_____
_____

DATE: _____

BREAKFAST:

At: _____ _____

_____

LUNCH:

At: _____ _____

_____

DINNER:

At: _____ _____

_____

SNACKS:
At: _____ _____

At: _____ _____

At: _____ _____

At: _____ _____

NOTES:

_____

_____

_____

_____

_____

WEIGHT: _____ *LBS*
              _____ *AM/PM*

DATE   TIME   BODY AREA

_____   _____   _____

EXERCISE	SET 1	SET 2	SET 3	SET 4	SET 5	SET 6
	REPS/LBS	REPS/LBS	REPS/LBS	REPS/LBS	REPS/LBS	REPS/LBS

CARDIO EXERCISE:

_____
_____
_____
_____

NOTES:

_____
_____
_____
_____

DATE:

_____

BREAKFAST:

At: _____

LUNCH:

At: _____

DINNER:

At: _____

SNACKS:
At: _____

At: _____

At: _____

At: _____

NOTES:

_____

_____

_____

_____

_____

WEIGHT: _____ *LBS*
                    _____ *AM/PM*

DATE   TIME   BODY AREA

_____   _____   _____

EXERCISE	SET 1	SET 2	SET 3	SET 4	SET 5	SET 6
	REPS/LBS	REPS/LBS	REPS/LBS	REPS/LBS	REPS/LBS	REPS/LBS

CARDIO EXERCISE:

_____

_____

_____

_____

NOTES:

_____

_____

_____

_____

DATE: _____

BREAKFAST:

_____
At: _____
_____

LUNCH:

_____
At: _____
_____

DINNER:

_____
At: _____
_____

SNACKS:
At: _____
_____
At: _____
_____
At: _____
_____
At: _____
_____

NOTES:

_____
_____
_____
_____
_____

WEIGHT: _____ **LBS**
                _____ **AM/PM**

DATE _____   TIME _____   BODY AREA _____

| EXERCISE | SET 1 | SET 2 | SET 3 | SET 4 | SET 5 | SET 6 |
	REPS/LBS	REPS/LBS	REPS/LBS	REPS/LBS	REPS/LBS	REPS/LBS

CARDIO EXERCISE:

_____
_____
_____
_____

NOTES:

_____
_____
_____
_____

DATE:

_____

BREAKFAST:

_____

At: _____

_____

LUNCH:

_____

At: _____

_____

DINNER:

_____

At: _____

_____

SNACKS:

At: _____

_____

At: _____

_____

At: _____

_____

At: _____

_____

NOTES:

_____

_____

_____

_____

_____

WEIGHT:　　_____ **LBS**

　　　　　　　_____ **AM/PM**

DATE   TIME   BODY AREA
_____   _____   _____

EXERCISE	SET 1	SET 2	SET 3	SET 4	SET 5	SET 6
	REPS/LBS	REPS/LBS	REPS/LBS	REPS/LBS	REPS/LBS	REPS/LBS

CARDIO EXERCISE:

_____

_____

_____

_____

NOTES:

_____

_____

_____

_____

DATE:

_____

BREAKFAST:

At: _____

LUNCH:

At: _____

DINNER:

At: _____

SNACKS:
At: _____

At: _____

At: _____

At: _____

NOTES:

_____

_____

_____

_____

_____

WEIGHT: _____ **LBS**
               _____ **AM/PM**

DATE   TIME   BODY AREA

_____   _____   _____

EXERCISE	SET 1	SET 2	SET 3	SET 4	SET 5	SET 6
	REPS/LBS	REPS/LBS	REPS/LBS	REPS/LBS	REPS/LBS	REPS/LBS

CARDIO EXERCISE:

_____

_____

_____

_____

NOTES:

_____

_____

_____

_____

DATE:

_____

BREAKFAST:

At: _____

LUNCH:

At: _____

DINNER:

At: _____

SNACKS:
At: _____

At: _____

At: _____

At: _____

NOTES:

_____

_____

_____

_____

_____

WEIGHT: _____ *LBS*
              _____ *AM/PM*

DATE   TIME   BODY AREA

_____   _____   _____

EXERCISE	SET 1	SET 2	SET 3	SET 4	SET 5	SET 6
	REPS/LBS	REPS/LBS	REPS/LBS	REPS/LBS	REPS/LBS	REPS/LBS

CARDIO EXERCISE:

_____

_____

_____

_____

NOTES:

_____

_____

_____

_____

DATE:

_____

BREAKFAST:

At: _____

LUNCH:

At: _____

DINNER:

At: _____

SNACKS:
At: _____

At: _____

At: _____

At: _____

NOTES:

_____

_____

_____

_____

_____

WEIGHT: _____ *LBS*
                 _____ *AM/PM*

DATE   TIME   BODY AREA

_____   _____   _____

EXERCISE	SET 1	SET 2	SET 3	SET 4	SET 5	SET 6
	REPS/LBS	REPS/LBS	REPS/LBS	REPS/LBS	REPS/LBS	REPS/LBS

CARDIO EXERCISE:

_____

_____

_____

_____

NOTES:

_____

_____

_____

_____

DATE:

_____

BREAKFAST:

_____

At: _____

_____

LUNCH:

_____

At: _____

_____

DINNER:

_____

At: _____

_____

SNACKS:

At: _____

_____

At: _____

_____

At: _____

_____

At: _____

_____

NOTES:

_____

_____

_____

_____

_____

WEIGHT: _____ **LBS**

_____ **AM/PM**

DATE   TIME   BODY AREA

_____   _____   _____

EXERCISE	SET 1	SET 2	SET 3	SET 4	SET 5	SET 6
	REPS/LBS	REPS/LBS	REPS/LBS	REPS/LBS	REPS/LBS	REPS/LBS

CARDIO EXERCISE:

_____

_____

_____

_____

NOTES:

_____

_____

_____

_____

DATE:

_____

BREAKFAST:

_____

At: _____

_____

LUNCH:

_____

At: _____

_____

DINNER:

_____

At: _____

_____

SNACKS:

At: _____

_____

At: _____

_____

At: _____

_____

At: _____

_____

NOTES:

_____

_____

_____

_____

_____

WEIGHT: _____ *LBS*
              _____ *AM/PM*

DATE   TIME   BODY AREA
_____   _____   _____

EXERCISE	SET 1	SET 2	SET 3	SET 4	SET 5	SET 6
	REPS/LBS	REPS/LBS	REPS/LBS	REPS/LBS	REPS/LBS	REPS/LBS

CARDIO EXERCISE:

_____
_____
_____
_____

NOTES:

_____
_____
_____
_____

DATE:
_____

BREAKFAST:

At: _____
_____

_____

LUNCH:

At: _____
_____

_____

DINNER:

At: _____
_____

_____

SNACKS:
At: _____
_____

At: _____
_____

At: _____
_____

At: _____
_____

NOTES:

_____

_____

_____

_____

_____

WEIGHT: _____ *LBS*
              _____ *AM/PM*

DATE _____ TIME _____ BODY AREA _____

EXERCISE	SET 1 REPS/LBS	SET 2 REPS/LBS	SET 3 REPS/LBS	SET 4 REPS/LBS	SET 5 REPS/LBS	SET 6 REPS/LBS

CARDIO EXERCISE:

_____
_____
_____
_____

NOTES:

_____
_____
_____
_____

DATE:
_____

BREAKFAST:

_____
At: _____

LUNCH:

_____
At: _____

DINNER:

_____
At: _____

SNACKS:
At: _____

At: _____

At: _____

At: _____

NOTES:

_____

_____

_____

_____

_____

WEIGHT: _____ *LBS*
_____ *AM/PM*

DATE

TIME

BODY AREA

EXERCISE	SET 1	SET 2	SET 3	SET 4	SET 5	SET 6
	REPS/LBS	REPS/LBS	REPS/LBS	REPS/LBS	REPS/LBS	REPS/LBS

CARDIO EXERCISE:

_____

_____

_____

_____

NOTES:

_____

_____

_____

_____

0-595-30567-9

www.ingramcontent.com/pod-product-compliance
Lightning Source LLC
Chambersburg PA
CBHW061340280526
45784CB00001B/77